The
WRIGHT CHOICE

Your Family's Prescription For
HEALTHY EATING, MODERN FITNESS, & SAVING MONEY

Advance Praise

Randy Wright and David Tabatsky have succeeded in creating a book that not only instructs and motivates, it entertains! It's probably the most enjoyable book on family health on the market today. And the food is terrific!

Bruce Kluger
USA Today Board of Contributors

※

Every chapter of The Wright Choice *avoids negativism and rueful appraisal of our ever-expanding waistlines, and focuses on the psychological underpinnings of healthy living: love of family and self, understanding why we eat what we eat, and the importance of exercise. Those of us that deal with devastating neurological diseases know that the best therapy is preventive, and the best prescription for a healthy life is to prevent disease before it starts. This book encompasses what is best in modern medicine together with potential pathways for achieving the ultimate goal of disease-free futures.*

Stanley H. Appel MD
Director, Methodist Neurological Institute
Houston, Texas

※

Dr. Wright's book perfectly supports our theme—"Be Safe! Be Respectful! Be Responsible!" His prescription for good food, exercise, and community awareness offers our students and their families a terrific model for healthy living.

L. Gail Garrett, PhD
Principal, Los Angeles Unified School District

※

As someone professionally committed to healthy eating, I find Dr. Wright's prescriptions are perfect for American families. Randy is not only a doctor; he's a teacher!
　　　　　　　　　　　　　　　　　　　　　　　Donna Leonard
　　　　　　　　　　　　　　　Founder, Diet Gourmet and TruMeals

※

Mark Holley has created a perfect blend of recipes for today's busy families, incorporating healthy ingredients, which are easy to make, taste great and won't break your wallet.
　　　　　　　　　　　　　　　　　　　　　　　Chef David Cordua
　　　　　　　　　　　　　　　　　　　　　　　Houston, Texas

※

Dr. Wright has given me the help and self-confidence I need to handle the challenges I am facing since having a stroke. His book is consistent with the outstanding care I received from him and his entire staff: unfailingly committed, dedicated and highly professional.
　　　　　　　　　　　　　　　　　　　　　　　Jennifer S. Watson

※

For a busy working mom, creating a healthy lifestyle is my top priority and my biggest challenge. Dr. Wright's book offers quick and delicious recipes for people on the go like me who are ready to embrace healthy living and lower their risk of chronic diseases. If you are going to read and use just one book on proper diet and healthy lifestyle, this is The Wright Choice!
　　　　　　　　　　　　　　　　　　　　　　　Mandy Kao
　　　　　　　　　　　　　　　Vice-President, Titan Management
　　　　　　　　　　　　　　　　Founder, Mandy Kao Foundation

※

The Wright Choice *is easy to read, entertaining, and provides valuable information for those seeking a healthier life style.*
　　　　　　　　　　　　　　　　　　　　　　　Dr. Lee P. Brown
　　　　　　　　　　　　　　　　Former Mayor of Houston, Texas

Foreword by Paul Osteen, MD, Lakewood Church

The WRIGHT CHOICE

Your Family's Prescription For
HEALTHY EATING, MODERN FITNESS, & SAVING MONEY

RANDY WRIGHT, MD
DAVID TABATSKY

Featuring 50 Quick 'n Easy Recipes from Chef Mark Holley

InTouch Media Health Network

The Wright Choice is not intended as a substitute for professional medical consultation in matters of family health care, including physical examinations, nutritional counseling, and psychological assessments. Whenever appropriate, we encourage you to seek expert medical help and/or legal advice. *The Wright Choice* should be used only as a general guide and not as the ultimate source of information on matters of diet, fitness, and general health.

The author and publisher shall have neither liability nor responsibility to any person or entity with respect to any loss or damage caused, or alleged to have been caused, directly or indirectly, by the information contained in this book.

With regard to anecdotal scenarios *(According to Me)* and medical evaluations ("DocSpeak") included in the book, all names have been changed or left anonymous.

Copyright © 2011 by Randall Wright
All rights reserved. Printed in the U.S.A.
No part of this publication may be reproduced or transmitted in any form or by any means, electronic or mechanical, including photocopy, recording or any information storage and retrieval system now known or to be invented, without permission in writing from the publisher, except by a reviewer who wishes to quote brief passages for inclusion in a magazine, newspaper or broadcast.

Published in the United States by InTouch Media Health Network
P.O. Box 25410, Houston Texas 77265

ISBN: 978-0-9835447-0-8

Library of Congress Control Number: 2011908906

Illustrations by Edna Cabcabin Moran
Cover and Interior Design by 1106 Design

For Crystal

In loving memory of Silver Breaux, Sr.
The stroke he suffered was the catalyst
for healing millions of others.

All forms found in this book are available for downloading at our website:

www.TheWrightChoiceRx.com

Contents

Acknowledgments	xv
Foreword—Paul Osteen, MD, Lakewood Church	xix
Introduction—*A Healthy Heart Starts in the Mind*	xxiii

Part One
Creating a Vision for Good Health

1.	Self-Understanding	3
	Your Very Own Ball and Chain	7
	Up Close and Personal: A One-on-One Assessment	12
	Your Very Own Litmus Test	17
	Likes and Dislikes	24
	Defining Your Goals	26
2.	Back to Your Family's Future	31
	Know Your Family History	32
	Like Father, Like Son?	36
	Your Genealogical Health Chart	38
	Medical Myths # 1–4	42
	Embrace the Responsibility!	47

3. America's Obsession with Weight   51
   What is a Normal Weight?   53
   Body Mass Index (BMI)   55
   Medical Myth #5   57
   Throw Away Yours Scales!   59
   Your Family Food Diary   62

4. Why Do We Eat?   67
   The Psychology of Food   72
   A Basic Burger Breakdown   74
   The Truth About Twinkies   75
   What the Ingredients Really Mean   78
   Love of Self, Family, and Community   79

5. Are You Really Smarter Than Your Doctor? 85
   The Curse of Childhood Obesity   87
   The Teenager Syndrome   93
   Disease States Revealed   95
   Denial Is Also a Disease   110
   But I'm Tired! (The Struggle for Sleep)   111

Part Two
Understanding What Makes You Healthy

6. What Should We Eat? Carbohydrates 101   121
   Carbohydrates: Friend or Enemy?   123
   Simple and Complex—But Simply Sugar   124
   The Great Energy Providers   128
   Identifying Good Sources of Carbs   133
   Take the Whole-Grain Train   134

Contents

7.	*The ABCs of Protein*	143
	Where Does Protein Come From, and What Does It Do?	146
	Traditional Sources of Protein: Meat, Chicken and Fish	147
	Vegetarian, Vegan, and Macrobiotic Diets	149
	Medical Myth #6	149
	Invasion of the Shake People	154
8.	*It's a Fat Fat Fat Fat World*	159
	The Good, the Bad, and the Saturated	162
	Medical Myth #7	169
	Cholesterol: The Good, the Bad, and the Confusing	170
	Helping Your Kids Choose Wisely	175
	If You Can't Eliminate—Moderate!	178
9.	*It's All About Calories, Knucklehead*	181
	What's a Calorie?	182
	Why Math Matters	183
	How Many Calories Will I Burn Reading This Chapter?	186
	How to Count Calories	189
	Frequently Asked Questions	189
10.	*Vitamins, Supplements, and Fads*	193
	The Easy Fix	194
	Medical Myth #8	195
	Save Your Money—and Your Life	196
	Natural Remedies	204

What's Right for My Family and Me?	206
11. *Water Break!!!*	209
The Magic Elixir	210
What's That Stuff Coming Out of My Tap?	210
Bottled or Bust	212
Medical Myth #9	213
The Beverage Wars	216

Part Three
Dr. Wright's Prescription for
Busy Families On The Go

12. *Home and Away: The Economics of Family Health*	221
How to Read a Food Label	224
A Pantry Makeover	235
Smart Shopping	241
Surviving Restaurants	252
Economizing at Home and On the Go	260
13. *Healthy Meals Made Easy: 50 Recipes to Feed Your Family*	263
The Miracle of Planning Meals	270
From Breakfast on the Run to Lazy Brunches	280
A Lunchbox for School and the Office	302
Picnic Dinners and Weekend Feasts	332
Dad's Super Sunday Grill	358
A Three-Week Menu	367
14. *The Family Training Zone*	373
The Hidden Gym in Your Home	383

Pass the Paint Can and Other Family Games	386
The Dining Room Table Workout	388
Exergamming	393
Yoga, PIYOLET and Meditation	394
15. *Home Sweet Home*	405
Medical Myth #10	406
Welcome the Portion Police to Your Dinner Table	406
The New American Plate	407
Raising Food-Responsible Children	409
When Saying Grace Means Slowing Down	410
Conclusion—*A Call to Action*	413
Index	423
About the Authors	435

Acknowledgments

I owe a great deal of thanks to many people who have helped me along the way to making this book happen. First, I must thank my wife, Crystal, for her love and support. I would like to thank my Grandmother Mom-Mom for teaching me to always be nice to everyone. I would like to remember lovingly Grandmother and Grandfather Wright. I want to say thank you to my mother and father who taught me how to passionately follow my dreams and to never give up. I would like to thank Crystal's parent for their support throughout this entire process.

Mark Holley is a great chef, as you will soon discover. He has also become a great friend, and I thank him for his patience and support as I put him through the ordeal of meeting my strict standards for creating heart healthy food. I would also like to thank Patrick Blackman and William Thompson from PESCE for their extremely skilled assistance in the kitchen.

The Wright Choice

As if I wasn't lucky enough to have Mark on board, it's been my extreme good fortune to add Houston's best up-and-coming chef, David Cordua, to our culinary team, with recipes representing his family's many restaurants and through his general support bringing this book to the public.

Last but not least on the healthy food front, I owe a great deal of thanks to Anne Dubner, who tirelessly delivered nutritional advice and dietary knowledge in the most cheerful way I could ever imagine.

Many others played a vital role in bringing all this together. I cannot give enough thanks to Paul Osteen, MD for his time, support, and prayers for me through this process. I also own a great deal of gratitude to Fr. Chester Arceneaux for all his prayers, spiritual guidance, and encouragement. Thank you to Simone Metoyer, Kim Porter, Chef Bobo, Chef Mark Hawkins, Meghan Hall, Derrick Mitchell, and Roslyn Bazzelle, Tiffany Travis, Gabe Vega, Edna Morans, Ronda Rawlins, Michele DeFilippo and the rest of the team at 1106 Design, Jim Livesey, Sandy Lawrence, Chris Labod and Linda Roberts *for their expertise.*

Thanks to *all those who gave me their support, advice, and taste buds to ensure quality information and delicious food.* Those individuals include; Amanda Bedford, Reshanda Quintero, Alisa Smallwood, Patricia Chavez, Whitney Montgomery PA-C, Dwight Haas, Sharon Brown PhD, Morgan Wilson, Stefanie Schupp, Kenneth and Elizabeth Clay, Mark Banschick MD, Kevin Smith MD, Garfield Johnson MD, Jakeen Johnson MD, Garvin Davis

Acknowledgments

MD, MPH, Melenda Jeter MD, MPH, Anthony Brissett MD, Annette Brissett PhD, Marcus and Hedi Smith, Monica Mcneil, Roger Mcneil MD, Rachael Mcneil, Wayne Franklin MD, Felix and Keisha Phillips, Jerry Nash PhD, Sharla Schoonmaker, Leo Houston, Jessica Quinterras, The Royal Blue and White Family, Ainsley Todd, Devon Davis, Dustin Lane, Gordon Williams, Michelle Reed, Crystal Brown-Tatum, Jackie Brown, Charletta Lynn Barton, Gordon Wingate, Reginald Adams, Mandy and William Kao, Lisa Reyna, Tene Thomas, Berkely Arrants, Kofi Burney, Randy and Sue Sim, Michael and Tammy Harris, and the rest of Leadership Houston (specifically Class 28—the best class ever).

I also want to say thank you to my good friend David Tabatsky for helping me find my voice through this whole process. I am a blessed man for many reasons, but the biggest ones will always be my wife Crystal and our children.

Randy Wright, MD
2011

Foreword

Dr. Randy Wright has been my friend for many years. He is a respected member of Houston's medical community, a loving and attentive husband and father, and is someone who models what it means to live a healthy, balanced life. He practices what he preaches, and *The Wright Choice,* is an outstanding inspiration to help all of us do the same.

As a doctor, I have seen firsthand the devastating results of preventable diseases, many of which are the result of the cumulative effect of years of poor health choices. So often, these diseases result in a diminished quality of life, which can never be regained. And sadly, many of these diseases and their effects could be avoided by simple changes in diet and exercise.

After treating hundreds of patients with preventable health issues in his own medical practice, Dr. Wright created *The Wright Choice* out of a desire to help others live a better, healthier, and longer life. The writing is compassionate, conveying an urgency that should inspire us to change our lifestyle choices in order to prevent the devastation of disease.

The Wright Choice isn't an "instant fix" self-help book. Instead, it is a comprehensive resource to help you achieve a healthy lifestyle. It clears up some long-standing medical myths, gives you the basics upon which to create better habits, offers ideas for busy families on the go, and encourages you to develop a vision for a healthy life. It is educational and informative but easy to read and very practical.

In addition, *The Wright Choice* includes tools to help you start modeling a healthy lifestyle for future generations. As a parent, I know that children often replicate the same lifestyle habits and patterns of their mothers and fathers. That is why Randy writes, "The responsibility for our children's long-term heath prognosis lies with the adults at home who are their primary caregivers." *The Wright Choice* encourages you to "consider your family first" and take responsibility for teaching and modeling a healthy lifestyle to your children. I believe *The Wright Choice* is a book every family should read.

In a world filled with confusing information—from the latest and greatest diet, to exercise videos promising to revolutionize your health, from vitamins claiming they will keep you young, to foods that may harm us and our children—we must be vigilant to discern the truth amidst the deluge of media and advertising we face each day.

The Wright Choice offers a clear path to navigate through all of the confusion and arrive at a place where we can establish a healthy and sustainable lifestyle. *The Wright Choice* is our step-by-step guide to a better future.

Paul Osteen, MD
Lakewood Church

Introduction
A Healthy Heart Starts in the Mind

Being healthy does not depend as much on what you do, but why you do it. Each day, millions of people commit to working out more and eating better. Sadly, they often fall short of accomplishing their goal. Why? Is it because they started the wrong diet plan or chose an incompetent personal trainer? Probably not. The reason is most likely internal, because achieving optimum health doesn't start with choosing the right diet or exercise plan—as popular wisdom may tell you—it starts with why you chose change in the first place!

I often tell my patients that a "healthy heart starts in the mind," which doesn't necessarily imply a new diet, a gym membership, or a personal trainer. None of those will ever provide long-term benefits by themselves unless you choose to live a comprehensive, healthy life. That means recognizing the resources you already possess, defining clears goals, and organizing a plan to make them happen!

My focus is on the family because success is more likely if everyone at home shares a common goal. As a doctor, I have seen patients struggle to improve their health without the support of their spouse and children. We need to engage our kids from an early age, because we all know that childhood (and adult) obesity is a growing epidemic in America. The solution is not merely parents and schools telling their kids to get healthy. Parents must model healthy behavior by living it at home each and every day! This book will help you become role models for your children and give you great opportunities to enhance your quality time with them.

Why should you care about living healthy? How could you choose otherwise? If you're not sure, let's take a peek into the lives of the Wilson family, who may remind you of some folks you already know in your own neighborhood. The parents are doing their best to balance their kids' hectic schedules with their own work obligations and social commitments. Carol, a mother of three and a legal assistant, is experiencing weekly headaches and swollen feet, which get so bad sometimes she has to miss work. Her husband, Jim, a high school coach, is gaining weight rapidly and complaining of worsening digestive problems.

Although they do their best to manage money, the Wilsons are struggling to save enough money to purchase a larger home. When it comes to eating, they try to eat what they think is healthy. They order salad when eating out (but use too much dressing), give their kids plenty of milk (except it's not always low- or non-fat), and keep

Introduction

water bottles in their cars. But all too often, their health is sacrificed for convenience because it's just plain easier to settle for the drive-thru at a fast food joint than to park the car and get three kids organized inside a restaurant where they could enjoy a much more balanced meal.

When it comes to exercise, the Wilsons belong to a local gym, but by the time they get home in the evening and get the kids fed, bathed, and finished with homework, it's time for everyone to go to bed. As a result, exercise for Carol and Jim happens sporadically at best, and it's the same for their kids, who get PE at school (hopefully) twice a week at the most.

But let's not judge the Wilson family negatively. They are good people who clearly want the best for their kids, but like many of you, life on the go for today's family is—let's face it—too hectic and much too distracting.

It sounds like the Wilson family needs a break. Maybe so, but what they lack is a plan. Their situation hasn't occurred overnight, and if they don't address most of these issues very soon they could be facing some dire consequences.

Unfortunately, the Wilsons typify many American families who lack the basic knowledge and motivation to turn things around and get healthy. But it doesn't have to be that way! For example, when it comes to money, most people realize that without a responsible and reasonable plan you will never achieve your financial goals. The same can be said for your health. It's like your finances. If you're not realistic and don't plan ahead, you may go bankrupt!

This book offers you a road map for changing your personal and family lifestyle so that you can live a longer, more fulfilling life, and eventually retire with your health not only intact but thriving.

Why am I so interested in your health? It's simple, really. I am a doctor, specifically a neurologist, specializing in disorders of the brain and nervous system. My experience includes a cross section of advanced training in the fields of neurovascular diseases, genetic diseases, movement disorders, epilepsy, sleep disorders, and chronic pain management, just to name a few. I currently serve as the medical director of a neuroscience and stroke center as well as a stroke rehabilitation center, both in Houston, Texas.

Through daily contact with my patients and their families, I often hear the complaint that when people retire, they are too sick to enjoy the money and time that they have worked so long and hard to preserve. They feel shortchanged, and their "golden years" are not turning out to be so golden. Many of them are too sick to travel and their drug costs are more than they can afford. They wonder, "How could this happen to me? I was never sick a day in my life, until now."

Well, just like you shouldn't start planning for retirement a mere five years before you stop working, living healthy should not start only when something goes wrong and your life becomes seriously interrupted. Many people are struggling with health issues that could have been avoided in the first place, if they had only known more about basic nutrition, fitness, and the value of spirituality, and how to apply those principles to their busy lives.

Healthy living doesn't happen overnight. It comes from making a series of good decisions on a daily basis. Good health happens when you choose a bowl of raspberries instead of a chocolate cookie when responding to a midnight craving. Healthy living sustains itself when you decide to play soccer with your son for 30 minutes instead of watching TV. Choosing a healthy lifestyle means not giving up on your eating plan when you "mess up." Practice makes perfect, and honest effort usually yields positive results. So, if you make the right decisions (most) every day, you *will* get healthy—physically, emotionally, and spiritually.

It is my goal to steer you in the right direction on your journey to living better. This book will help you discover how a healthier lifestyle benefits every aspect of your life, from energy output at home and at work to less time and money spent on health care, from increasing your capacity to play with your children and love your spouse to decreasing your dependency on pharmaceutical drugs. It's all about making the right choices!

My prescription for you and other busy families on the go is not a miracle diet plan, and it is not designed to help you lose weight in a specific amount of time. It's not meant to give you super abs in ten days or your money back! This book is designed to serve as a lifelong guide to helping you (and your family) become as healthy as possible, while minimizing your chances for developing chronic medical conditions, such as high blood pressure, arthritis, or diabetes. You'll be pleasantly surprised to find out that once you are well on your way to following the principles in this book, including a host of new food recipes, you will most likely experience healthy weight loss and redistribution, but in ways that are sustainable in the long term.

Equally, or in some cases more important, this book will ask you to evaluate how you, your spouse, and your children operate together as a family unit. Being a religious man, I find immense value in spiritual teachings. They encourage us to question our lifestyle while challenging us to be our best. Regardless of our faith, each of our bodies should be seen as a temple and must be treated with respect.

But that can happen only by putting what you learn into positive, concrete action. The opportunity to do that lies right here within these pages, through information, advice, and recipes. Call it a prescription for better health to inspire you, your spouse, your children, and your community. Somewhere down the road, once you've begun to experience the benefits of applying these principles to your daily lives, we invite you to share your stories on our website. The improvements you make at home will also inspire others to do the same.

Today's world is ultra-competitive and, in many ways, harsh and inconsiderate. We need to be strong and resolute, and as parents, it is our job and God's calling to be

Introduction

positive role models for our children. We are what we eat, where we play, and how we behave. We must live our lives with mindfulness and with hope, and it all starts at home, with our families, one day at a time.

I sincerely hope that this book will help you realize that nourishing your family's health is the most essential thing you can strive for, and that it's your responsibility to do your utmost to achieve and maintain it. Without good health, all the money in the world will mean nothing. Learning about what constitutes good health and how you can actively guide your family in that direction is a noble effort, and one not to be taken lightly. Look around your neighborhood and community. You'll see evidence that once people take personal responsibility for their health, many good things will fall into place.

In parts one and two of this book, we will explore the psychology of eating, evaluate your health, and learn exactly what it is that you are putting in your bodies. Through simple facts and figures, you will come to understand the truth about carbohydrates, proteins, fats, and calories. Once you know these basic principles, it will be time to take on a new set of behaviors in part three, featuring a comprehensive food plan, a guide to making your home a healthier place, and an enjoyable game plan for family fitness.

Imagine if you could create a Family Bill of Health and post it on your refrigerator for everyone to see on a daily basis. What would you include? Perhaps you could start with your right—and obligation—to be educated and responsible for your family's good health. Specifically, you might agree not to feed your children anything you wouldn't eat yourself. But why stop there? How about pledging to make your dinner table family friendly, share your thankfulness for your lot in life, and promise to pay attention to each other each and every day?

Remember, a healthy heart starts in the mind. And there's no better time to start changing your life than right now.

Part One

Creating a Vision for Good Health

CHAPTER 1

Self-Understanding

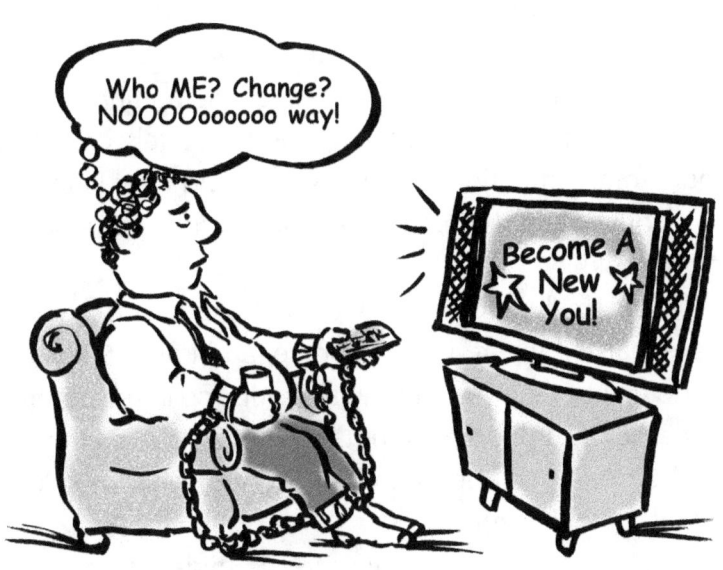

What About You?

Most people have bad habits. For example, I don't get enough sleep, I exercise infrequently, and I eat on the run way too often. Sound familiar? Those are three bad habits right there. But I'm working on it!

All kidding aside, if you saw me, I would appear on the outside as a picture of good health. I'm slim, youthful enough (nearing forty), and appear to have zero health issues. In a country obsessed with weight and flat tummies, I would appear to be in excellent health. But upon closer inspection, I could probably stand to gain a few pounds, increase my muscle tone, and reduce the puffiness under my eyes by getting more sleep. And I definitely could pay much more attention to what, when, and how I eat.

You're right. I am an excellent candidate to read my own book!

One small point: I am aware of my erratic behavior. I have learned where I can improve, and I am on my way to doing just that. I would say that puts me in the minority because most people are not paying very good attention to their own well-being or, I'm sorry to say, the overall health of their family.

How about you? Are you in the midst of improving your health? Or are you stuck in some version of the same old, same old? If so, why? Do you understand your true value? Are you really comfortable with who you are right now and where you see your life heading? What about your spouse and your kids?

Can you conceive of defining your goals? Are you ready to become healthier and happier? If so, you're ready to benefit from this book. If not, you can continue reading, keep an open mind, and take this opportunity to conquer your old habits. Because the sooner you identify your weaknesses and make the necessary changes, the sooner you can begin living a more energetic, productive, and fulfilling life.

WARNING!

Do Not Keep Reading If You Do Not Intend to Improve Your Health.

STOP!
EXERCISE BREAK!

This book is dedicated to improving your family's health.

You are reading it right now because you're interested in doing that.

We applaud you for making this choice.

Setting the right example starts with you, as an adult member of your household.

So, before reading any further, please put down this book, choose your favorite exercise, and do it for at least five minutes.

Five minutes!

That's all (for now).

Just take five minutes—out of a total of thirty minutes for the day and make that each and every day, of course, as recommended by the American Heart Association.

Ready?

If you can't decide on an exercise, go to Chapter 14, where you'll find some great ideas to get you started.

What are you waiting for?

It's only five minutes!

Your Very Own Ball and Chain

The elephant is a colossal being that can stand ten feet tall and weigh up to 11,000 pounds. These powerful creatures have the power to uproot trees and level buildings. However, once in captivity, these powerful forces of nature behave quite differently. If a young elephant is tied to a tree with a chain, it soon finds that it cannot break free. The baby elephant will try and try to escape, but it soon learns that its efforts are futile and gives up. Over time, as the elephant grows, the chain that once kept the baby elephant from escaping its prison becomes no match for the powerful adult animal. However, something interesting happens; the elephant that has been held in captivity all those years does not try to break free even though it has the physical capacity to do so. The elephant has been conditioned to believe that it cannot escape and accepts being bound by the same small chain, which held it as a baby.

Just as the mind of the elephant can be conditioned to believe in things that simply are not true, so we as human beings can be conditioned to limit our abilities. This "baby elephant syndrome" may also be called the "learned helplessness syndrome" and is well described in psychology literature. This syndrome gives great insight into how we as humans are often trapped by experiences in our past.

How many times have you tried to do something new but fell short on your first try and then told yourself that you knew you would fail, because you've always done so in the past? The good news is that humans are different than elephants, and we possess the ability to move beyond our past experiences. We can choose a different path if we really want to. All of us are blessed with a mind and the capacity to reason, and we have the power to change our future by not being bound to our past.

I raise this point because developing a vision for your health means not dwelling on past negative images, but looking forward to where you desire to be. Many of the patients I treat say they want to live a healthier life, but when we dig deeper, they really believe that being overweight is just their lot in life. They have seen their parents, grandparents, and several other family members struggle with weight, and subsequently they internalize that problem as their own.

According to Me

I went to see Dr. Wright because I couldn't sleep. I snored terribly, had constant headaches, and I was tired all the time. He asked me all these questions about how I felt about myself, what I was eating, and how much exercise I was getting (none). I really didn't want to talk about all of that because I was kind of depressed and didn't feel like anything could change. I realized later that I hadn't done anything to help myself, but I guess I was just too scared to change.

Jamie, age 31, Houston, Texas

Self-Understanding

The first step on the path to a healthier you—and a healthier family—is to break the chain of poor self-confidence.

"DocSpeak"

Jamie had a condition called obstructive sleep apnea, which results from obstructed breathing during sleep. It can cause excessive daytime sleepiness and frequent headaches. Treatment usually involves sleeping with a machine called a CPAP (Continuous Positive Airway Pressure), which provides a flow of compressed air designed to keep a person's airway open. People with obstructive sleep apnea are often overweight, so in addition to treatment with CPAP, I often discuss weight loss and exercise. Jamie was no exception. As we explored her activities, it became apparent that Jamie's view of herself was not very high. She didn't seem very confident in her ability to make a significant change in her life. At each visit, she would casually report that she had tried to eat better and exercise more, but for one reason or another, she was never able to follow through. Even though she knew she needed to make these changes, Jamie just couldn't seem to get it together.

What is it that holds many of us back from doing what we know we should do to live healthier lives? Looking inward can help us answer that question. Our self-image is an important factor in what we are able to achieve. Individuals with poor self-esteem often find it difficult to accomplish any significant tasks.

As you read about Jamie and contemplate your own situation, are you in any way doubting your own potential for following through on your goals?

According to Dr. Mark Banschick, a noted psychiatrist and author of *The Intelligent Divorce*, self-doubt is a natural phenomenon, but it only becomes a debilitating factor if we let it cripple our forward movement into uncertain territory.

"People like Jamie can be overwhelmed with shame and it stops them from taking proactive steps to get healthy. Whenever Jamie feels ashamed about her weight, she thinks about something else and feels better, at least temporarily. If she considers going to the gym, where she'd compare herself to others, Jamie anticipates the embarrassment, so she doesn't go. Her sleep apnea problem presents a similar dilemma: knowing that her weight makes it worse, Jamie feels—what else—shame.

Because shame is just a feeling, based on a mistaken belief that you are weak or unworthy, you must objectify it and don't let it win. This is why life coaches, therapists, dietitians, and personal trainers can be so helpful. They hold you accountable to that part of your mind that wants to be healthy and holds your shame at bay. Once new habits take shape, shame has a way of dissipating."

The process of developing a healthy self-image starts in childhood. Raising your self-esteem in regard to living a healthier lifestyle is rooted in understanding that your existence is important, and that you have a special role to play in this world. A lot of us undervalue our lives and

Self-Understanding

treat ourselves accordingly. You have to see yourself as God sees you: unique and with purpose in this world.

Paul tells us in his letter to the Corinthian's: "Don't you know that you yourselves are God's temple and that God's spirit lives in you?"[1]

Father Chester Arceneaux, currently the pastor of Cathedral of St. John the Evangelist Parish in Lafayette, Louisiana, gathered extensive experience in relationship counseling while serving his former students at the University of Louisiana.

When I spoke with Father Arceneaux about self-esteem, he reminded me of what Psalm 139 reveals: "God made each of us with a special purpose. God often uses those who seem unlikely or unworthy in the world's eye to accomplish great tasks. This is important to understand for we all are important in God's eyes, and no matter what our current condition may be, God loves us and has a special purpose for us."

Father Arceneaux cited some of his students as examples, advising them to learn a more disciplined approach, and to see how smaller accomplishments over time help build confidence and give us the strength to tackle larger tasks.

As Father Arceneaux suggests, if we see ourselves as God sees us, we will know that our future is bright, and we are well equipped to accomplish any task. The limiting factor is not necessarily based on skill, but on our self-image!

---

[1] 1 Corinthians 3:16

My former patient Jamie's inability to make the needed changes in her life was not because of any physical incapability; it was because she was psychologically unable, which likely stemmed in part from a low self-image. Before I could realistically expect her to succeed with any eating or exercise plan, I had to help her realize her true value and that her health was important not only to her, but to her entire family.

This applies to anyone wishing to shake off poor habits and negative thoughts and live a healthier lifestyle. While some of us may not subscribe to a formal god, each of us has the power to find the proper motivation for improving our lives. Most likely, you will discover that in the faces of your spouse and your children.

Up Close and Personal: A One-on-One Assessment

Self-esteem affects your daily habits and, inevitably, your health. Once you honestly assess how you feel about yourself, you are one step closer to improving your overall well-being. But before you can make any kind of significant life change for yourself and your family you must first examine your motives and determine your readiness.

When you look in the mirror, do you admire the person looking back at you? When all of your friends have gone home and you have stopped boasting about all the push-ups you did this morning, does a little voice in your mind say, "Hey, you really should start working out, ya know?"

Self-Understanding

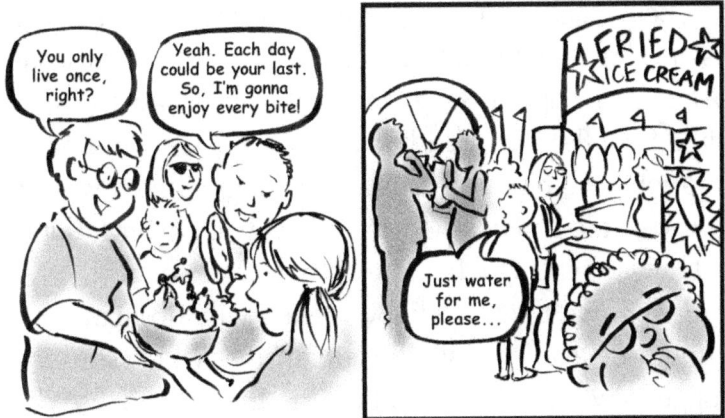

Have you ever been at an 8 a.m. company meeting and grabbed a sugarcoated pastry instead of the fruit, saying to yourself, "I know I should have the fruit, but I really need energy and something to fill me up this morning."

Or have you ever gone to your son's Little League game and ordered a steamy, sloppy chili cheese dog, thinking to yourself that one little hot dog couldn't hurt, even though you actually do the same thing every week, at every game, throughout the season?

Practice What You Preach and Preach More Practice

Very few of us live the healthiest life we can. I know I don't. There. I said it. But many of us know, at least in principle, what we need to do to be healthy. The problem comes with putting our thoughts into action.

Before I go any further, let me confess something. When I started writing this book, I could do only three push-ups before giving up, laughing. Then I realized it wasn't so funny. Little by little, I kept adding to my total, and I'm now up to about one hundred a day, including a bunch with my two-year-old son on my back. I don't want to brag, but I'm actually practicing what I preach! What a concept!

So, if we think we know better, why do many of us cringe, or even get slightly defensive, when someone suggests we should eat fruit or skip the chili cheese dog? Why is it that so many of us can offer what seems to be a reasonable explanation for what we eat and what physical activities we engage in, but on closer inspection seem questionable, at best? How can we be so good at fooling ourselves?

Education, Awareness, and Denial

Many people are not aware of the consequences of their actions when it comes to their health, and they feel that their actions do not put them at risk for problems down the line.

D-E-N-I-A-L.

Are we even aware of it while it's happening? Regardless, it's time for all of us to stop living in denial and pretending not to care. We all want to live long and productive lives. I have treated many patients who have told me similar stories about how they looked forward to retirement and put off certain trips or activities until they reached that point in their lives. But once they reached retirement, they were too sick to do anything and felt

Self-Understanding

like they were getting a raw deal out of life. They spoke about how they thought they would have time to travel the world, eat exotic foods, and spend endless hours playing with their grandkids.

Their reality, however, was much different. Strokes prematurely disabled many of them. Obesity limited the movements of others because of chronic pain syndromes. Heart disease claimed the lives of many spouses, leaving their survivors alone to face the world. High blood sugar levels left many disabled, unable to travel or enjoy a good quality of life.

Each story is heartbreaking and eye-opening. I have learned so much from my patients, and this is why I am sharing their life lessons with you. The truth is, some of the conditions and diseases that have limited many of my patients' ability to enjoy their golden years are actually preventable!

We can no longer eat food blindly, thinking only about how it tastes and makes us feel. We must take into account how food can help or ruin our bodies. Education is the key, and this book will provide you with the knowledge you need to recognize your current situation and make the right choices for you and your family. Filling the awareness gap is the easier of the two problems. The more difficult problem to tackle is our almost innate tendency to deny that problems exist, and to act on them once they are recognized.

According to Robert Surles, aka Chef Bobo, a graduate of The French Culinary Institute, Executive Chef and

Director of Food Services at The Calhoun School in New York City, and author of *Chef Bobo's Good Food Cookbook,* "The best way to educate kids about healthy eating is by feeding them real food that has been well prepared. To me, healthy food equals real food (not processed food). Real food is prepared using ingredients that are natural and fresh."

Sounds simple enough, doesn't it? So, why not get started? The first step is to honestly assess your current knowledge and habits. This will give you a starting point from which to measure improvement. The goal of this book is not just to educate and entertain you, but to literally walk you, step by step, toward improving your health and your family's, too.

Self-Understanding

Your Very Own Litmus Test

Let's find out what you already know and what you're about to learn. Write down your answers here in the space provided, and once you've read the rest of the book, you should have a perfect score.

1. Does your grandmother's health play a role in your well-being?
2. If you think you feel fine, should you still bother seeing your doctor?
3. What weighs more, muscle or fat?
4. What's in a fast-food burger?
5. How many children in America are obese?
6. What's a carbohydrate?
7. Where does protein come from, and what does it do?
8. What is trans fat?
9. How many calories should I eat, on average, each day?
10. What is in a multivitamin?

You and your doctor should have already figured out the answers to questions 1 and 2, and if not, what are you waiting for? Put down the book and make an appointment! Meanwhile, you can find the rest of the information in Chapters 3 through 10.

Right now, let's go a step further, so you can find out more about you.

The Wright Choice

Life Style Assessment

KEY: Never = 0   Sometimes = 1   Always = 2

1. Do you exercise at least 30 minutes a day?
2. Do you smoke?
3. Do you see a doctor on a regular basis to check your vitals?
4. Are you aware of your daily calorie intake?
5. Do you eat at least four servings of fruit and vegetables daily?
6. Do you eat at least six servings of whole grains daily?
7. Do you choose lean cuts of beef, pork, or other meats?
8. Do you eat salmon at least twice weekly?
9. Do you avoid eating the skin of meats and chicken?
10. Do you remove visible fats from the meats you eat?
11. Do you drink fat-free or low-fat milk?
12. Do you eat fewer than five servings of sweets weekly?
13. Do you actively seek out low-salt foods?
14. Do you avoid fried food?
15. Do you avoid foods with partially hydrogenated fats, trans fats, or saturated fats?

Self-Understanding

16. Do you drink low-calorie beverages?
17. Do you have no more than one alcoholic drink daily (women) or two or less daily (men)?
18. Do you have a pre-planned, weekly grocery list?
19. Does you spouse share your goals for healthy eating?
20. Do you have a sit-down meal with your family at least three times per week?

ASSESSMENT
A higher score indicates a healthier lifestyle.
A lower score points to a lifestyle that needs serious changes.

With these two simple tests, you now have a starting point from which to measure yourself as we move forward. If you have high scores on both the knowledge part and the lifestyle portions, this book will provide you with helpful tips and practical plans to maintain long lasting health. If you scored poorly on both the knowledge test and the lifestyle assessment, then the upcoming pages will provide you with eye-opening information that will enhance your understanding of personal and family health and how your actions can literally change your life.

If you scored high on the knowledge test and low on the lifestyle portion, you may either be in denial or having difficulty managing your behavior. Join the club. You obviously know what you should be doing, but have not put your knowledge into practice.

The Wright Choice

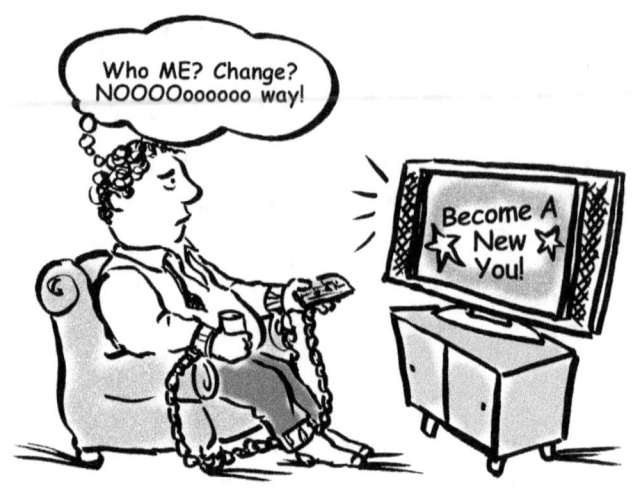

This book will show you how to take what you know and incorporate it into a manageable program, taking into account your busy schedule.

Finally, if you scored low on the knowledge test but high in the lifestyle portion, then although your intuitions have proven to be good, imagine how much healthier you can become when your choices are based on solid information and proven formulas for better living.

Moving forward, we will start from the ground floor and build a foundation for good family health. Chapter by chapter, you will learn what's needed to make the choices that will create an optimum situation for you and your family.

Motives

The first step in any journey is to know where you are going, and why. Many people claim that they want to lose

Self-Understanding

weight, but why? Do they simply want to look sexy to attract a certain person? Do they want to be the envy of all their friends? Or is it because they want to live a healthier life, and they know that weight loss will be a key factor in attaining that goal?

What's your motive for buying this book in the first place? Curiosity? Interested in losing weight? Lowering your blood pressure? Easing arthritic pain? Inspiring your spouse to get off the couch and get in shape? Are you determined to become a role model for your children?

Whatever the reason may be, understanding your fundamental purpose is critical to your success and anyone else's that you may be including in your journey. It's simple. We must define our personal and family health objectives and then devise a plan to reach our goals. Merely saying, "I want to lose weight" is not enough to succeed in your quest for long-term weight management. In order to create any meaningful and lasting experience, we must seriously question our motives and come to a clear understanding of why we are doing something before we start. Then we must set simple and specific goals—and the more specific, the better. If we don't do this, we may get lost in the process and end up quitting early or getting distracted to try something else.

More important, we must be patient and willing to practice! Reaching our goals will take time and patience, and practice is always necessary.

Let me suggest a motive that I consider applicable to most any situation. We all know the expression, "as long as we have our health." It's true. When we're healthy, everything else has a better chance of falling into place. Couple that with the desire that every parent has for his children—health and happiness.

With these common denominators in mind, we are all in the same boat.

What better motive could there be than bringing your family together in an atmosphere of good, sustainable health and authentic happiness?

Motivators

Now that we understand the importance of defining our mission, we must take stock of ourselves and acknowledge our personal assets and liabilities. Only then can we lead our families on the right path.

Preparation, attention to detail, and a passion for what we are doing are three key elements for success.

Every morning, the operating rooms in hospitals all across America are bustling with activity, long before any surgery begins. At the crack of dawn, anesthesiologists arrive to do a visual inspection of the patient they are about to put to sleep for surgery, and they assess the machines they will use for those purposes. This is done with meticulous accuracy, taking into account the size of the patient's mouth, the depth of her throat, and a thorough review of her entire medical history. Then they review the surgical plan to determine if any potential problems exist that may result in rescheduling, or even cancellation. Once the patient is cleared for surgery, the

Self-Understanding

anesthesiologist inspects the anesthesia machines again, verifies that the medications they will need are available, and makes sure the operating room staff is ready.

The anesthesiologist takes all of these steps because he or she realizes that failure is not an option. He is responsible for the life of the patient during the operation. Nothing must go wrong, and if something does, the anesthesiologist must be prepared to deal with it. While I am not suggesting that adjusting your diet, learning to exercise, and bringing your family together are life-and-death matters (at least in the short term), we should prepare like any anesthesiologist does for the journey we take with our body and spirit, if we want to afford ourselves the highest chance for long-lasting success.

All too often, we jump into things without really knowing what we are getting into. For example, some people start jogging as their primary mode of exercise, without taking into account prior knee problems, and soon quit because of recurring pain and frustration. How many times have you joined a gym, but soon realized that you could not get there on a regular basis, because your daily schedule did not afford you the time? How many diets have you started only to quit because the food you were asked to eat did not fit your budget or was extremely different from what you normally ate? Taking stock of our lives before embarking on a journey is always a wise choice, if we really want to succeed. Preparation is key.

Taking stock of your current health and state of mind is an important step in your journey to a healthier lifestyle.

Start with your doctor and get a complete physical exam. Identifying problems like high blood pressure, diabetes, arthritis, or even heart disease are important conditions to identify before making any significant lifestyle change. Getting the blessing from your primary care physician with regard to increasing physical activity is helpful in preventing unintentional problems down the line.

After undergoing a physical assessment, understanding your psyche is the next step. This may sound simple, but many people skip this phase and miss out on engaging in meaningful activities. It's vital that you are realistic about the goals you wish to achieve.

When I first started working out, I followed the usual pattern; I went to my local gym and signed up! I loved the gym; it was close to work and had great hours. The only problem was, the last thing I wanted to do after completing hospital rounds at 7:30 p.m. is spending a hour in the gym and getting home close to 9 p.m. to a tired wife with two little children! After assessing what was important in my life, understanding my time constraints, and taking into account the obligations I had to others, I realized that having simple exercise equipment at home worked best for my family and me. (In Chapter 17 we'll introduce a few ideas for equipment you can also have in your home.)

Likes and Dislikes

There are many ways to live a healthy lifestyle, and throughout this book we'll explore these options in great detail. At this point, I want to underscore the importance of thinking

Self-Understanding

about your likes and dislikes, because these will dictate which path to good health works best for you and your loved ones.

For example, I love being home with my family, so I try to be there for as many meals as possible, and my wife and I try to make them family centered. It's good for our two little boys to learn this model from the very beginning. I exercise at home, sometimes with my kids (imagine my son urging me to do more push-ups!), and I make sure to organize family outings as often as possible.

But I need something more organized. With a busy schedule, I don't want to count on luck and random availability. I know that the only way I will really get to do these things I love is to focus, write things down, and make them happen.

On a daily basis, it's relatively simple, really. Many of us write things down so we don't forget to do certain errands on our way home from work or while we're driving cross-town to pick up our kids from soccer practice.

I do that, too, like everyone else, but my *To Do List* reflects much of what I want to do about getting healthy. For example, I remind myself constantly about doing 30 minutes of rigorous physical activity every day. (More on what constitutes "rigorous" in Chapter 15.) I also jot down reminders of what I want to cook for my family at least three times a week, and also to actually stop racing around and sit down and enjoy a nice, slow dinner with them at least three days every week. Feeling positive about these things makes it a whole lot easier to anticipate achieving them.

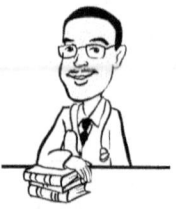

THE WRIGHT ADVICE

Make a *To Do List* and practice following it.
As I mentioned, I've got my own agenda for becoming healthier.
I'll feel better in the short and long run, and
more than likely my wife will, too.
Not to mention that I'd like to continue
running around at top speed
with my two growing children.

Defining Your Goals

While a *To Do List* is intended to help us focus on our short-term, daily issues, we can all benefit by establishing a goal chart to address the bigger pictures in life. You may want to refer to your two assessment tests for inspiration.

My Goal Chart is focused on the bigger picture of my life and the welfare of my family, now and down the road. It's designed for success but it's much more important than a simple *To Do List* because it's aimed at a long-term vision for where I want to get and how I want my family to get there with me. Understanding what needs to be done and following through in a way that works for you will deliver lasting results.

Self-Understanding

Consider what you're doing to plan ahead for your retirement. The key thing is you have a plan. If you want to be healthy enough to take advantage of your retirement, you need to create a vision for your good health. It's not all a question of chance. Not at all! You can control a lot of your physical and emotional well-being.

Confucius once said, "Choose a job you love, and you will never have to work a day in your life." Donald Trump has echoed this theme more recently, as he teaches eager entrepreneurs to find what they love to do and turn that into a business. This also holds true with regard to finding the path to a healthier life. If you can enjoy the things you do, it is easier to continue doing them.

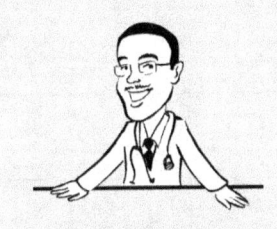

RANDY'S RULES
Be realistic about setting goals.
Be patient.
Set your sights just a little bit higher.

MY LONG-TERM GOALS

Please use this space to write down your long-term goals.

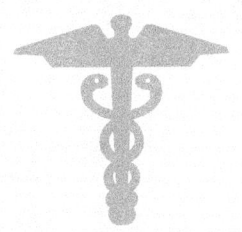

The Wright Reminders

Be honest with yourself.

Challenge your family to get healthy.

Identify your motives and motivators.

Make a To Do list.

Put your thoughts into action.

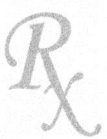

CHAPTER 2

Back to Your Family's Future

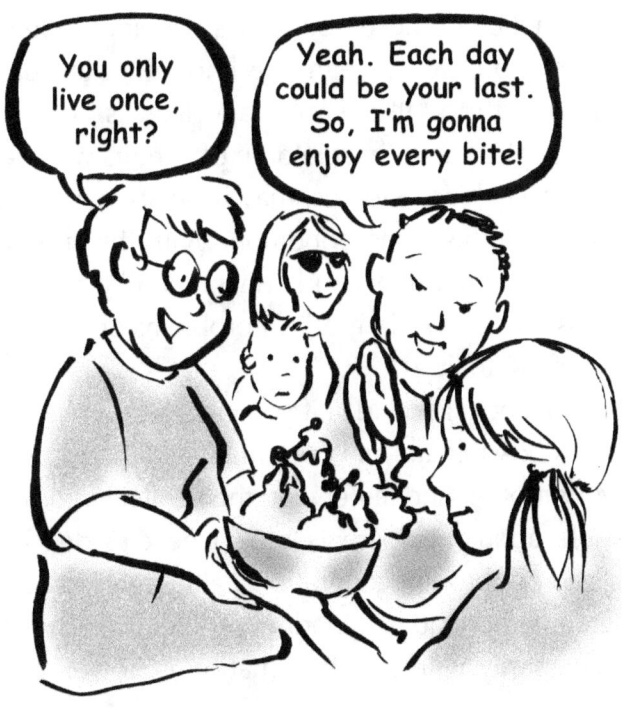

Know Your Family History

When seeing a doctor for the first time, he or she may ask you many questions in order to understand your background and the nature of your illness, if that is the reason for your being evaluated. Questions range from past medical conditions to current symptoms and usually include queries about any medical problems that run in the patient's family.

Recording a thorough family history is a powerful tool for medical student training. It has been long understood that many medical problems run in families. The role of genetics in these conditions is being understood more and more every year. We know that tall parents often give birth to tall children, and likewise for shorter individuals. We know that children of parents with certain conditions, such as diabetes, may have an increased risk of developing this same condition. With this in mind, it becomes easier to understand how our family history may predispose us to certain medical problems or physical (or even mental) abilities.

It would be a good idea if you gathered as much information as possible about your family health history. Start with your mother and father, and then collect information, if possible, about their parents, too. Genetic tendencies can be passed on through generations, although just because your grandfather had gall bladder problems doesn't mean you necessarily will, too. Information is power, and the more facts you can provide for your physician, the better diagnosis he or she can give you in return.

Once you establish your own family facts, fill in what's relevant for your spouse. Include all the details you possibly can. Some day, this information will become relevant and useful for your children.

According to Me

Growing up as the middle child among five siblings, with two seemingly healthy parents and two sets of grandparents, I never questioned whether there might be any illnesses running in our family. But as I got older and found out about one grandmother's diabetes, another's worsening arthritis, and one grandfather's struggle with cancer, I began to wonder. The same year I graduated college, my mother was diagnosed with breast cancer, but at the time, I never asked any questions about our family. About five years later, I gave birth to my first child.

The next Thanksgiving, we were all together, except for my grandfather, who had passed away. Two of my brothers also had new children, and one of my sisters was pregnant. My mother was ailing but no one said a word. During that dinner, while feeding my daughter, I realized how little I really knew about my family. As a new mother, I felt that it was my obligation to take care of myself and be healthy for her. I started asking questions right there at the table. My siblings joined in, eager to know. My parents and grandparents, reluctant at first, ended up sharing a tremendous amount of information, as well as beautiful memories. When I returned home after the weekend, feeling closer to everyone, I made an appointment to see my doctor and have a breast exam.

Brenda, age 42, Duluth, Minnesota

"DocSpeak"

Brenda has certainly done the right thing. Growing up with a seemingly healthy family around her, she made a typical mistake assuming that everything was okay and that she didn't have anything to worry about. Luckily, by the time she became a mother, Brenda had figured it out. Unfortunately, most families have a history of some kind of illness or disease, but family members either don't share important information or don't ask, and as a result they aren't in the best position to help themselves.

As a neurologist, I am constantly trying to tap into my patients' family histories, and any information they provide is potentially useful.

According to the United States Department of Health and Human Services, 96 percent of Americans believe that being informed about their family health history is important, yet only a third of those people have actually gathered together that information and written it down.

In 2004, the Surgeon General declared Thanksgiving to be National Family History Day. Why don't you make it your chance to find out more about your family and help yourself and your loved ones along the way? Remember, if you don't act like Brenda and go see your doctor to find out how things may affect you, you've gone only part way toward ensuring your own good health.

Like Father, Like Son?

Have you ever thought about your family's health history and how it may be affecting your lifestyle decisions, and those of your current family? Have you noticed that many families have children proportionally similar to one of their parents in size? Those children may also have similar taste in clothing (at least when they're little!) and may share similar tendencies with hairstyles, walking gaits, and speech patterns.

Are all these things genetically determined? Some may be, but the role of what scientists call "nurture" is often just as important. This "nurture" is all the habits and ways of doing and thinking that we learn from our parents and our environment. These behaviors are not necessarily hardwired, and may be altered. So when we are looking at making lifestyle changes, it's helpful to understand why we do some of the things we do. Growing up in certain cultural and ethnic circles exposes us at an early age to develop preferences for food, a certain level of physical activity, and specific behavioral patterns.

I grew up in Louisiana, where sitting down and eating several pounds of crawfish on the Fourth of July was what people did. I didn't realize that barbecue was an alternative until I moved to Texas. Those born and raised here in the Longhorn state often gasp at the thought of eating "mud bugs" instead of a good steak, especially on big holidays.

Our upbringing and cultural backgrounds play a big role in shaping our behavior as adults. Without realizing it, we may take certain things for granted as healthy endeavors, such as greasy barbecues, roasted marshmallows, and an endless supply of sweet tea and sugary lemonade. While these habits are certainly breakable, knowing our family health history is equally important because it can play such a vital role in developing a plan of sound preventative care as we grow older. In some cases, we may even be able to break the chain of disease! Knowing it is one thing; how you can change it is quite another!

STOP!

EXERCISE BREAK!

Even if your family doesn't have a history of exercising, it's time for you to get started creating your own legacy.

Go ahead.

Just five minutes (at least for now), and then back to reading the rest later.

Your Genealogical Health Chart
(To be filled in for each parent)

Father

Father's Father

Father's Mother

Siblings

Children

Paternal Grandfather

Paternal Grandmother

Maternal Grandfather

Maternal Grandmother

Your Genealogical Health Chart
(To be filled in for each parent)

Mother

Mother's Father

Mother's Mother

Siblings

Children

Paternal Grandfather

Paternal Grandmother

Maternal Grandfather

Maternal Grandmother

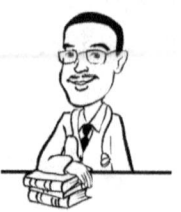

THE WRIGHT ADVICE

The Internet offers plenty of helpful medical sites, but nothing replaces the give and take you can experience with your general practitioner.
I urge you to make an appointment with your doctor to see how you can modify your lifestyle before developing any serious problems.

Are You As Healthy As You Think?

I've spent years teaching others about the keys to healthy living. I have spent many hours preparing lectures and developing material to be used by others in their quest for better health. I have seen many patients in my clinic, over multiple visits, discussing eating plans and exercise routines, only to discover at subsequent visits that they had not stuck to their plans. Why? Why do people who know what they are supposed to do simply not do it? The answer is obviously complicated and differs from person to person, but there are some common threads.

First, let me ask you this question: Is your health gauge accurate?

Do the things you attribute to being unhealthy truly reflect your health?

Back to Your Family's Future

Consider your automobile. Most people have a lot of experiences with cars, and to me, there are many analogies that can be made between cars and humans. Take the various gauges on a dashboard, for instance. There are many gauges that tell you about the health of your car. We trust these gauges to be accurate, because if they aren't, we won't be warned in time to deal with these problems that are easily foreseeable.

For example, you would have a gauge problem if you ran out of gas while your gas gauge still read that your tank was half full. Most people would be pretty angry if this happened, because it would lead us into an unfortunate situation where we could be stranded, or worse still, cause some kind of permanent damage to our car. Running out of gas should be an avoidable problem. Gas is normally very easy to get before we run out; all we need is to be adequately warned by our gas gauge. If this were to happen to you while driving a long distance, it may lead to anger, confusion, and distrust in the other gauges in your car.

Because you ran out of gas when you really weren't expecting to it can lead to lots of unexpected expenses and an awful experience. Besides that, you would not get to where you intended to be (certainly not on time), and you wouldn't reach your goal on an empty tank of gas. That's not to mention what could happen if you were using low-octane gas in a car that requires high-octane fuel.

But all of this could have been avoided if the gauge in your car was working correctly. Just like a malfunctioning gas gauge can lead to major problems with your car, so can a faulty personal health gauge lead to your own poor health.

Medical Myth #1
"I feel great. Therefore, I must be perfectly healthy."

Unfortunately, I have heard the same line from patients over and over again: "Doc, I've been healthy my whole life. I never saw a doctor, ever, and now you tell me I just had a stroke."

Many people measure their health by how they feel and pride themselves on never having to run to a doctor. This perspective is very common, but unfortunately it's a very dangerous one to maintain.

"If I don't have any pain, I must be healthy."

All to often, people evaluate their own health in terms of perceived pain. They figure an absence of pain means an absence of disease. The problem with that thinking is many conditions that put you at risk for major health complications do not hurt. High blood pressure is called "the silent killer" because it is a major risk factor for heart disease and stroke, yet it carries essentially no signs or symptoms, in and of itself. High cholesterol and even diabetes are chronic diseases (we'll cover them in detail in Chapter 11) that are usually painless at first, but if not treated early on can eventually lead to devastating and painful consequences.

Let's return to the example of our car. If you hear a noise while driving and your car isn't operating properly, you know you better take it to the shop and get it looked at and fixed. You might've already learned your lesson the hard way, after ignoring the last noise until you found yourself stranded on the freeway with a stalled engine or a flat tire. So the next time you heard something fishy, you didn't hesitate and drove straight to the garage. More than likely, the mechanic knows more than you do, and he or she will tell you what is wrong and what is needed, whether a part needs repair or replacing. As long as you trust your mechanic, you'll be relieved to know that your car will be up and running again very soon.

The first lesson is, when you noticed something not working right, you did something to take care of it before it got worse. You fought off the urge to deny the problem and overcame any impulse you may have had to be lazy and put it off for another day—when it may have already been too late.

The second lesson you can learn from taking your noisy car to the mechanic when you did is something altogether deeper and not always so obvious. That is, when you noticed something not working right, the damage is likely already done and it is time for a repair. The question is, could that repair have been avoided in the first place?

What about maintaining your own body, as you do your car?

If you notice a problem, say, chest pain, for example, and the doctor tells you that you have blocked arteries, the fact that you have something wrong should not be a shock, especially if you have never had routine checkups.

Just like the car dealer recommends periodic checkups, including basic oil changes, tune ups, etc., we humans also need regular maintenance, especially as our "mileage" increases.

Waiting to see a doctor until we have problems is not the best way to lead a healthy life. Many of the illnesses we suffer from as a society can be avoided if we take a proactive and preventative approach with our lifestyle.

We shouldn't wait until our arteries are clogged before going to the doctor and then wondering "why me" and being upset that life was unfair. Small steps of prevention can make a huge difference in long-term health. Unlike a car, because doctors are not the master engineers, some problems can only be managed, and simply replacing a part or fixing the root cause is not always an option.

The best treatment is prevention, and regular doctor visits are highly recommended.

Medical Myth #2
"My parents and grandparents were overweight, so being overweight is normal, right?"

Wrong! Humans come in different sizes, and variation is good. God made us all unique, so there is no one mold we must fit into physically. However, it is well described in medical literature that obesity can shorten life and lead to many chronic diseases, such as heart disease, stroke, diabetes, sleep apnea, and chronic pain. The list goes on and on. In fact, according to the Center for Disease Control,

90 percent of our country's health-care costs are related to obesity.

We will go into detail about the dangers of obesity in Chapter 5, but I cannot stress this fact enough: obesity is a dangerous medical condition.

Individuals and family members should recognize it as such, and that just because everyone in your family is obese, that is no reason to consider it acceptable, let alone a healthy option. More important, there is still hope for all of you to shed a few pounds.

Medical Myth #3
"I'm thin, so I must healthy."

Wrong again! Weight is not the main measure of health. I know I just stated that being overweight is unhealthy, so it should stand to reason that being thin, or at least close to your ideal weight, is automatically healthy, right? Wrong! Not all diseases that affect us are linked directly to weight. Infections, cancers, some forms of arthritis, epilepsy, and many others have nothing to do with weight. So don't be overconfident if you are a lean and mean machine; you still need regular checkups with a physician.

"But I like how I look in a bathing suit. What else is there to worry about?"

Vanity is a great seducer. When we let our appearance be our only gauge for health we may be setting ourselves up for unnecessary problems.

It can work both ways.

Focusing on losing weight to look good is not a fair measure of health. A reasonable perspective on weight is important. We all want to look good when we hit the beach, when all eyes are on us. That's fine; it's a natural desire. But when the only reason we diet is to achieve a certain body weight just to look good in a bathing suit, problems usually develop. First of all, we must realize that our weight results from the balance of fats, muscle, bone, and other body tissue. Some of these structures we can manipulate to get weight down, but others we cannot.

There are many ways to manipulate one's weight: crash diets, starvation, vigorous exercise, etc. Most people who engage in weight-altering activity for the sake of appearance rarely maintain long-term health. Many of the fad diets are not sustainable and people either quit because of inconvenience or are taken off the diets because of health complications.

We must change our perspective on weight and its relationship to our overall health. This will be a steady topic for discussion in subsequent chapters.

Medical Myth #4
"All I need to do is take the pills my doctor gave me, and I'll be okay."

Too often, patients stop listening once they receive a prescription for medicine. Imagine a doctor prescribes antibiotics for a nasty chest infection and the patient walks out of the office, feeling like it's just a matter of time before he'll be feeling fine again. He celebrates by having a cigarette in the parking lot.

Once you have asked your doctor any questions you deem necessary about his or her recommendations, and you feel comfortable with the diagnosis, then I do encourage you to take what your doctor prescribes. But you would be wise to use the occasion to review your normal health habits and reconsider what behavior may have contributed to your illness in the first place.

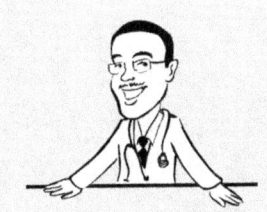

RANDY'S RULES
See your doctor at least once a year.
If you don't have a doctor,
put this book down right now and get one!

Embrace the Responsibility!

That is not the end of the story. We all bear responsibility for our own health. Doctors can do only so much to help keep you healthy. Most of the responsibility for one's health is in the hands of the individual. In addition to taking medications as prescribed, we must also lead lifestyles that promote health.

Using our car example again, if you want to keep your car for a long time, you don't want to drive it too hard. You have to take care of your car for it to take care of you. If you abuse your car, it will not run for long.

Same with our bodies. If we abuse them or simply don't give them the simple attention they need, they will soon wear out on us. Take responsibility for the one and only body God has given you!

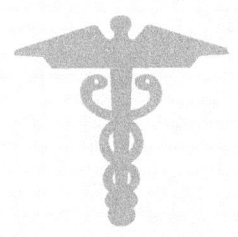

The Wright Reminders

Fill out your family health chart.

Identify risks.

Assess your current state of health.

Ask your doctor to help you.

Embrace the responsibility.

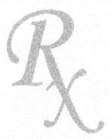

CHAPTER 3

America's Obsession with Weight

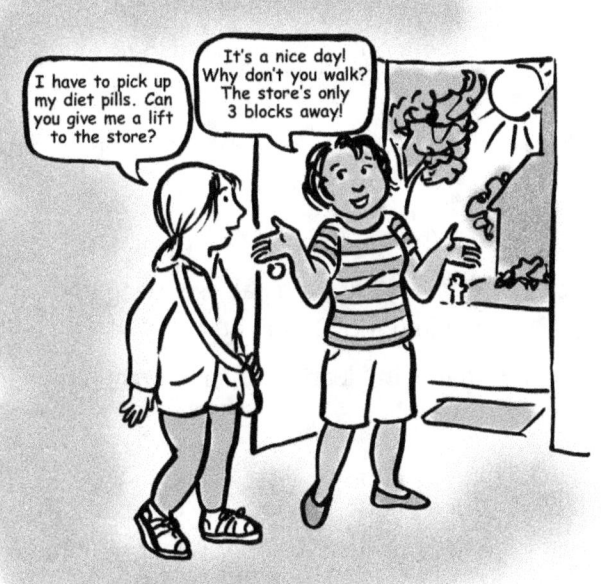

"How Do I Look?"

You can't turn on the television anymore without being assaulted by shows like,
The 50 Million Pound Challenge, The Biggest Loser, or *Kirstie Alley's Big Life.* Not to mention the endless amount of commercials hawking diet programs, exercise equipment, and weight-loss medication.

> **STOP!**
>
> **EXERCISE BREAK!**
>
> Speaking of television, most of us
> watch entirely too much of it,
> which reminds me—we need to exercise.
> You should have the routine down by now.
> Five minutes or more (for now) and keep reading!
> Wait.
> Why not jump to ten minutes?
> After all, we're eventually shooting for a
> minimum of 30 minutes each day,
> as the American Heart Association recommends.

Let's face it. Our society has become obsessed with weight. People will go to unbelievable lengths to lose it, but it doesn't seem like anyone is asking why so many people in our country are obese in the first place. I don't want to put anyone on television out of work, but can you imagine if we weren't a country with so many overweight people? Can you picture a TV program that millions of people tuned in to each week where they could learn how to get healthy before it was too late and they gained all that weight? Why don't any of those television programs share even one little hint about how its viewers, home on their couches, munching away on snacks, could put down the calories and do a bit of exercise while they're watching the weight-loss programs?

In fact, it's the media that shapes much of our distorted view of what is healthy and attractive, as well as what we perceive to be proportionally correct. America's obsession with weight is all too often twisted by an unrealistic vision of "perfection"—perfect abs, perfect breasts, and perfect teeth—all virtually unobtainable by the average person but relentlessly displayed as necessary for success and to be desired by all. For decades, Madison Avenue has hijacked our common sense, and I hope that many of you reading this book will come to a more reasonable conclusion.

What is a Normal Weight?

For now, let's consider a reality each of us can control. In spite of the perverse amount of advertising we encounter on a daily basis, baiting us to spend our money on fads and get-skinny-quick schemes, there is a substantial amount of truth to the claims that many of us need to question our current behavior and take steps to get healthier.

Following is a statement many patients fear hearing when they go to the doctor.

"Please step up on the scale and let's take you weight."

It seems that the only measure of health people pay attention to these days is weight. In many cases, it's a word that is feared. While a person's weight certainly plays a very important role as an indicator of general health, I fear that the underlying meaning of weight has been lost in all the marketing to promote weight loss. An individual's weight has become the Holy Grail for determining one's health.

We previously discussed four medical myths, which have adversely affected the way people gauge their health. While weight is certainly not a false gauge, I think it is one that is often misunderstood and taken out of context. So let's spend a little time discussing weight and how we can analyze it properly.

What is a normal weight? This seems like an easy question, but in reality it's a little more complicated. Weight is more that a number on a scale. It is an indirect measurement of nutritional status. However, weight alone is an incomplete assessment of nutritional states. Our ideal body weight is a function of height and changes accordingly. A measurement that calculates our height and weight is called the Body Mass Index (BMI). It's one of three tools for assessing whether someone is overweight, along with waist circumference and other risk factors for disease and conditions associated with obesity, including high blood pressure, high cholesterol, high blood sugar, and diabetes.

According to a National Heart Lung and Blood Institute (NHLBI) study, almost 108 million American adults are overweight or obese. If you are one of these people, carrying this extra weight puts you at risk for developing many diseases, especially heart disease, stroke, diabetes, and cancer. Losing this weight helps to prevent and control these diseases. The NHLBI guidelines provide you with a new approach for the measurement of overweight and obesity and a set of steps for safe and effective weight loss.

The statistics indicate that more than one third of the adult population is either overweight and/or obese. Those numbers may be even higher now, ten years later. The ramifications are staggering. The burden this puts on individuals, families, and communities cannot always be measured in finite terms, but consider how many potentially productive days are lost because people are sick and missing school, work, and important events as a result. Consider the labor that life can become when you are carrying around a significant amount of extra weight.

The National Institute of Health and the American Heart Association have established guidelines to determine what is healthy. I follow many of their recommendations and will be sharing them with you throughout this book. Let's look at their evaluation methods for determining if our height and weight are those of a generally healthy person.

Body Mass Index
Underweight = <18.5
Normal Weight = 18.5–24.9
Overweight = 25–29.9
Obesity = BMI of 30 or greater

The Wright Choice

According to the Department of Health and Human Services, the National Institutes of Health's National Heart Lung and Blood Institute and Obesity Education Initiative, obesity and being overweight substantially increase the risk of morbidity from hypertension, dyslipidemia, type 2 diabetes, coronary heart disease, stroke, gallbladder disease, osteoarthritis, sleep apnea and respiratory problems, and endometrial, breast, prostate, and colon cancers. Higher body weights are also associated with increases in all-cause mortality.

That's a devastating list. I face those issues every day at the hospital. My hope is that some of you reading this book right now will eventually take yourselves off the list of potential fatalities and get yourself and your families on the road to better health. Each chapter of this book will give you key facts and figures to help you do just that.

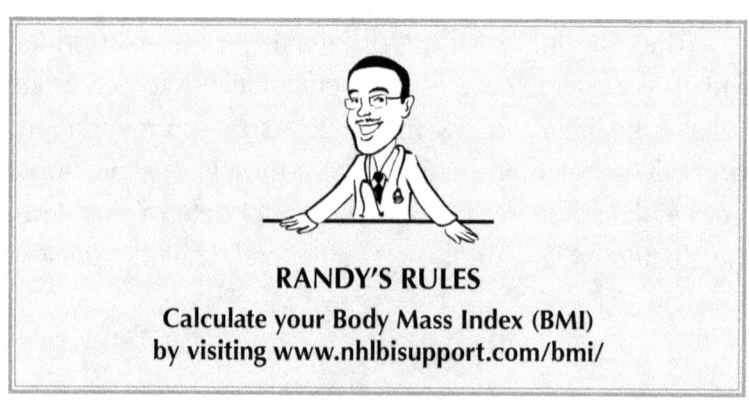

RANDY'S RULES
Calculate your Body Mass Index (BMI)
by visiting www.nhlbisupport.com/bmi/

Medical Myth #5

"If I gain any more weight, I'm gonna die!"

The leading cause of death in America is cardiovascular disease, NOT being overweight. Those of you who are health savvy may argue that our (measured) weight is an entity that we must fear and fight feverishly to control. Virtually every fitness magazine and health book, along with a barrage of television and Internet information, has launched an all-out war against being overweight. The media seems to be catering to our inner ego, making us believe that being thin and beautiful is the most important marker of health.

If you ever have the chance to review death certificates, you will almost never see the cause of death as being overweight. Death in most cases is related to cardiovascular disease (heart attacks, congestive heart disease, and even stroke). While excessive weight may lead to any of these conditions, being overweight, by itself, is not the problem.

The real issue is the cause. Some people are simply affected by genetics and are born with a natural inclination for adding weight. But some may have normal, healthy cholesterol numbers, stable blood pressure, and no signs of heart problems. If they eat well (as we will define in Chapters 12 and 13), get regular exercise (Chapter 14), and approach life with a positive attitude, they should continue to live healthy lives. That being said, those people who are predisposed through their family history to be overweight should pay extra attention to the risks that extra weight can often present. It's no secret that overweight people are at greater risk for a host of problems.

> **According to Me**
>
> I always see these overweight actors in the movies and on TV who run around, jump off buildings, chase people, and generally look like they're in such good shape, even though they could stand to lose a whole lot of weight. How could they do all that? Whenever I see somebody big doing something like that, I figure I am overweight, but why can't I do that stuff, just like those actors? How hard can it be? After all, I saw it on TV. It must be real.
>
> *Bruce, age 44, Dayton, Ohio*

"DocSpeak"

I'm a doctor, not an actor, but I do know that actors get lots of second chances when they're filming a television show or making a movie. Then again, and this is crucial, they are actors, pretending to be in good health, when probably they're not. Entertainment is built on illusion, and while actors are meant to fool us into believing they are other people, often acting out fantasy lives onscreen, in reality it's quite a different story. In fact, many actors have died tragically because they abused their bodies, either through drug and alcohol addiction, overeating, or a host of other reasons.

Bruce, like many others who watch too much TV, has a hard time distinguishing between what is real and what is an easily created illusion. As a doctor, I can only hope he will come to his senses and get the help he needs to overcome his weight issues.

Throw Away Your Scales!

Today's prevalent thinking identifying weight as the enemy we must fight to live long, healthy lives is simply inaccurate! I see my patients jumping on diet bandwagons every day, only to fall off within days or weeks because they are trying to lose weight for the wrong reasons.

We are inundated with diet plans and workout schemes that focus on short-term goals. As a society, we are generally short-term minded. We all want quick fixes and instant results. Sadly, many people would rather take a pill to lose weight, ignoring the potential side effects, rather than make the lifestyle changes that address weight issues and improve overall health.

Don't let the scale control your life. As you gain muscle through exercise (like weight lifting) and lose fat from aerobic workouts, the scale may not show much difference from your starting point. That's because you're trading unhealthy weight (fat) for muscle. One pound of lean muscle has less mass than one pound of fat. So while the numbers on your scale may not budge, you will notice your clothing fitting differently, as well as that extra bounce in your step.

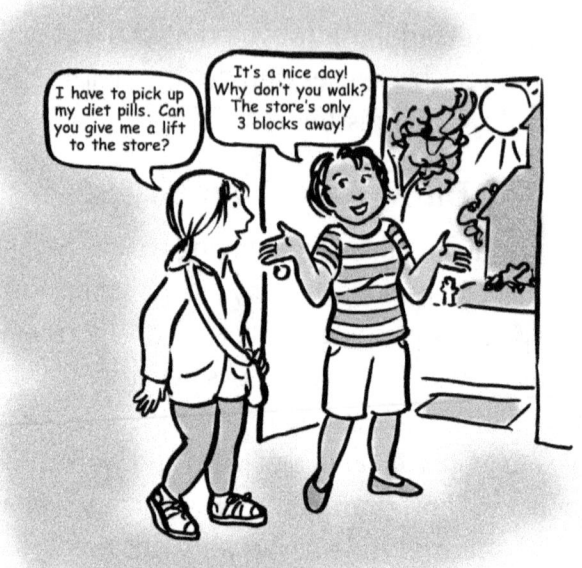

Who Are We Fighting?

A good analogy in our ongoing battle with weight is the wars we are fighting in Iraq and Afghanistan. Suicide bombings and ambushes on our soldiers are horrible events and should be stopped. So the question arises: Should our war generals focus the war on identifying every potential suicide bomber and stopping them before they activate a bomb? Should the main goal of our mission be to find all the enemy soldiers in hiding and attack them before they ambush us?

If we did that, we would most likely see a reduction in the number of suicide bombings and military ambushes in the regions we attacked, but would that really indicate that we had won the war?

No. Because the individuals who are the masterminds behind the bombing attacks will simply change tactics. The war will continue, and our efforts, though valiant, will ultimately be ineffective. The problem was, we did not go after the root cause of the attacks. We went after the foot soldiers and not the generals. To win a war, we have to understand the enemy and not focus our efforts on battles that will give us only superficial, temporary victories.

A friend of mind told me something that completely identified the problem many of us have when we think about health and weight. He has high blood pressure and was exercising and trying to "eat right" to improve his health. He had read a few magazines and knew about watching his intake of carbohydrates.

With that knowledge in tow, he ate in the hospital cafeteria where he worked. He got a hamburger and proudly did not eat the bread because of its carb content, but ate just the meat because beef is low in carbs. AAAAGGGGHH! My well-informed, intelligent friend threw away the bread, which has carbs with no real nutritional value, but NO trans fats. Instead, he ate a piece of meat—institutional, I might add—filled with trans fats that will contribute negatively to his ongoing atherosclerotic process (clogging blood vessels, a problem we'll discuss in detail later) that leads to high blood pressure and eventual heart disease.

This seemingly educated but unfortunately misinformed approach is what many people are taking when it comes to their eating choices. We are fighting the foot soldiers and letting the masterminds go free. If we continue this habit for too long we will ultimately lose the war.

So how do we determine who the masterminds are, what their plan is, and how we can counter those plans and win the war?

First, you must identify exactly what you and your family are eating on a daily basis, including snacks, late-night indulgences, and food on the go. Only when you look closely at your current habits can you even consider changing them for the better. Here you will find a ten-day chart we suggest you fill in with every detail possible. Later in the book, we will analyze some of its content and you will see how easy it is to figure out where you can begin making improvements.

Your Family Food Diary

The chart on page 64 is meant to help you document everything your family eats over a period of ten days, including the extra portion of pasta you wolfed down at the last minute, or that glob of dressing you poured over your salad. Not to mention the snacks you eat while driving. It's so easy to forget all the things we eat while we're on the move throughout the day. But it's vital that we do because all of them can really add up to an amazing amount of calories.

"But it's just a bite here and there."

"I didn't even eat the whole bar."

"What's the big deal? It was a small soda!"

"My daughter didn't finish her mac and cheese. I can't just throw it away."

"I was busy watching the news. I didn't even realize I ate another one."

Sound familiar? Gotcha! Me, too. Let's not even talk about the empty calories I've eaten while working on this book. One of America's biggest pizza chains has been trying to convince us that a basic slice of pizza has significant nutritional value. I have to admit that sometimes, while working long hours, I became so hungry I almost believed them. All kidding aside, I really do watch what I eat but I slip up just like everybody else.

I'm convinced that the best, and only, solution is keeping a food diary (next page), which you can also download from our website (www.TheWrightChoiceRx.com). Once you've filled in everything—and we mean everything—it will be easy to identify your eating habits and determine where and how you can make changes, individually and as a family.

The Wright Choice

Family Member Name _____

	Breakfast	Lunch	Dinner	Snacks
DAY 1				
DAY 2				
DAY 3				
DAY 4				
DAY 5				
DAY 6				
DAY 7				
DAY 8				
DAY 9				
DAY 10				

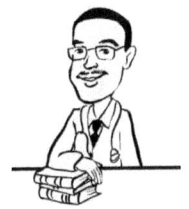

THE WRIGHT ADVICE

We believe in the power of community.

When you visit
www.TheWrightChoiceRx.com
you will find much more than charts, tables, and helpful facts.

You will meet other people who are committed
to creating healthier and happier families.

We welcome your thoughts on all the topics covered in this book and hope your feedback will help to inspire others.

Some of your ideas may appear in the next version.

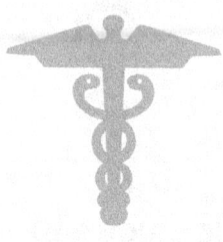

The Wright Reminders

Have your BMI measured at your doctor's office.

Throw away your scales.

Pay attention to everything you eat.

Make a family food diary.

Exercise!

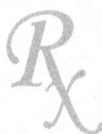

CHAPTER 4

Why Do We Eat?

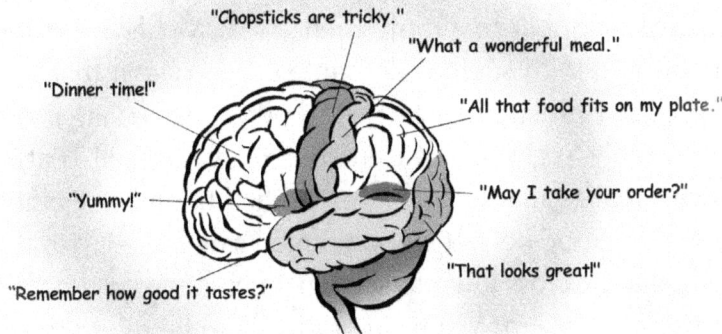

Thoughts on Food

"But it tastes so good."

Sitting at the dinner table with my wife and close friends is always a pleasure. We enjoy the great company, stimulating conversations, and, of course, the fabulous food. Sitting in a restaurant, you cannot help but be mesmerized by all the mouth-watering options.

Warm rolls and breads start the meal. The sweet smell of freshly baked bread beckons your nose to come closer. This tempting introduction is soon followed by a host of appetizers that seem to make your palate and stomach leap for joy. This is soon replaced by utter amazement as the main course is served. It seems that great food is such a relief to the soul that all your pains, worries, and stressors appear to simply melt away. Meals are often associated with such a pleasant social context that it is difficult to remember that the real purpose of eating is not necessarily to give us pleasure, but to give us fuel! That is, until I realize that I eat on the run half the time, wolfing down my food between appointments or while I'm in the car, racing across town to see a patient in the emergency room. In those moments, I eat merely to fill my stomach so I won't be distracted by hunger while I'm supposed to be concentrating on something more important. Or I eat simply because it's such a familiar thing to do.

I must admit that I don't always make good choices about what I eat. All too often, I opt out for the easy picks, avoiding healthier alternatives simply because they're not available at the drive-thru. After all, purchasing better food means pulling over, getting out of the car, and maybe even waiting in line when I'm in a hurry. Fast food is much easier, right? I mean, it's a no-brainer, isn't it? Maybe not. In the long run, maybe I should be asking myself, what's so comfortable about comfort food, anyway?

Life demands that we pay better attention to why we eat. Certainly eating on the run is not healthy. It usually means we're eating fast food (or something close) and even in a nice restaurant we could be ingesting extremely fatty foods (because they taste good) that are essentially just as bad as a greasy burger. Why do we keep repeating the same habits, especially when they aren't healthy?

According to Me

My mother was forced to move to Arizona to live with me after Hurricane Katrina completely devastated her home. The southwest presented a shocking physical change for her. The air was dry and she had less connection with the water than she did living off the banks of the Mississippi River.

In New Orleans, food was the glue that kept most families and communities together. My mom was constantly cooking fried shrimp dinners, crawfish etouffee, and fried oysters for her church parish, her friends, and family whenever they were around. Everyone loved her cooking, but they loved her stories even more. She loved to sit on the porch in her rocker, recalling how it was growing up in New Orleans.

But all of that changed for my mother—twice: the first time was when the hurricane hit, and her life was turned upside down a few years later when she had a heart attack.

After a lifetime of eating fatty foods and lots of greasy meat, my mother has modified her gumbo recipe to include much less salt and butter, very little meat, and she now incorporates brown rice into her daily diet. We walk together every day and my mom has actually gotten me to live more healthily, as well.

Marcy, age 37, Scottsdale, Arizona

"DocSpeak"

Marcy's mother was lucky. She was given a second chance—twice! Her story is the essence of what many Americans experience. Our lifestyle is woven into our culture. In my home state of Louisiana, food is life and relationships are everything. However, those southern traditions have also spawned some unfortunate habits. In fact, that region, which includes Alabama, Arkansas, Georgia, Indiana, Kentucky, Louisiana, Mississippi, North Carolina, South Carolina, Tennessee, and Virginia, is often referred to as "the Stroke Belt." That stems from its exceptionally high rate of cardiovascular-related diseases, including heart attacks and strokes. So while many may adore the culture, there is plenty of room for improvement when it comes to preparing great-tasting food that is healthy.

Marcy's mother, despite her good intentions, learned that lesson the hard way. Behavior, as well as genetics, plays a major role in health. Just like she heeded the warning signs of Hurricane Katrina and left before the storm hit, had she listened to the warning signs her body was giving her, she may have been able to avoid having a heart attack. It seems as if her daughter, Marcy, has heeded those lessons and is modifying her lifestyle to become healthier.

The Psychology of Food

Sustenance—feeding ourselves for health and survival—is the main reason why we eat. Scientifically, it's the only explanation. Culturally, of course, it's an entirely different ball game. I mean, eating alone can be fine but sharing a meal with loved ones and friends can be a meaningful experience, on many levels. So if you prefer to eat with people you care about (including yourself), then shouldn't you be caring about the food you eat?

First, consider your family. Is it really okay to give them junk? One fatty meal may not be so dangerous, or a sugary treat, or a stadium hot dog, but if you eat all three of those—and we all know too many people are doing just that—you are putting your health at serious risk, especially if you eat like that on a regular basis. It's like parking your car (here we go again) outdoors through a snowy, wet winter. Eventually, the underside will rust and rot and fall apart.

You may not have a choice where you park your car, but you can control what you eat. Would you ever tell your husband or wife to walk across the street blindfolded, risking a serious accident? I'm sure you wouldn't. Could you imagine sending your children to school in shoes that hurt their feet? I doubt it. So why is it so easy to serve our loved ones a plate of food that may be harmful to their health? I'm guessing the simple reason people keep making bad choices is because they don't know what's in the food they're buying, cooking, and serving.

Why Do We Eat?

Let's fix that. Remember that Whopper? And the Twinkie and the hot dog? You'd be amazed how much you're compromising your health when you eat just one of these—once.

"Fast food and junk food are very difficult habits to break," says Robert Surles, author of *Chef Bobo's Good Food Cookbook*. "In this way they are like other addictions. They appeal to our hunger for salty, crunchy, sweet, and fatty foods. Plus, they are easy to find and cheap to purchase."

You say you can't help it? You feel like you've just got to indulge? Same with your kids, huh? They bug you and you just can't help giving in? What's one more little piece of junk food, right? You almost have our sympathy because we understand how persuasive the advertising industry can be when it comes to convincing you to purchase certain food products—for you and your kids. The Grocery Manufacturers Association spends more than 1.6 billion dollars per year alone advertising an assortment of junk food. Their ads are aimed directly to kids, and they try to hook them when they're very young. It's no wonder that it takes a tremendous amount of willpower to withstand the onslaught of commercials aimed at getting you to buy more and more and more!

But you can make the right choice! Perhaps it will help if you know more about that junk food that seems so tempting.

A Basic Burger Breakdown
aka
The Whopper Revealed

Serving size	1 sandwich Whopper 290 g Jr. 158 g
Calories	670 Jr. 370
Calories from fat	350 Jr. 190
Total fat	39 g Jr. 21 g
Saturated fat	11 g Jr. 6 g
Trans fat	1.5 g Jr. 0.5 g
Cholesterol	115 mg Jr. 50 mg
Sodium	1120 mg Jr. 570 mg
Total carbohydrate	51 g Jr. 31 g
Dietary fiber	3 g Jr. 2 g
Sugars	11 g Jr. 6 g
Protein	28 g Jr. 15 g
Source	www.BK.com

Why Do We Eat?

Equal Time for the Big Mac

Serving size 216 g	Calories 590	Calories from Fat 306
Total Fat 34 g	Saturated Fat 11 g	Cholesterol 85 mg
Sodium 1070 g	Total Carbohydrates 47 g	Dietary Fiber 3 g
Sugars 8 g	Protein 24 g	

The Truth About Twinkies

A Twinkie is described as a "golden sponge cake with creamy filling." It's four inches long and is a golden color with a dark caramel-colored base. It has three puncture marks on its underside where the white creamy filling has been inserted. If you eat enough of them, you could end up with puncture marks in your chest from bypass surgery. In case you're not convinced, consider a Twinkie's ingredients, a veritable Top Ten list of unfortunate and forbidden foods, including:

(1) corn syrup (2) high fructose corn syrup (3) corn syrup solids (4) animal shortening (5) beef fat (6) sodium stearol lactylate (7) artificial flavors (8) food coloring yellow 5 and red 40 (9) modified corn starch, and last but not the least unhealthy (10) Polysorbate 60.

Each Twinkie contains 2 g of saturated fat, 20 mg of cholesterol, 2000 mg of salt, 25 g of carbohydrates (of which 14 g is sugar), 1 g of protein, and absolutely no fiber at all.

The Wright Choice

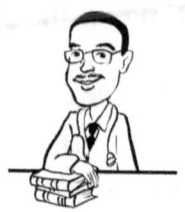

THE WRIGHT ADVICE
Stay away from Twinkies and other snacks masquerading as food.

Sure You Want That Hot Dog?

Serving Size: 1 hot dog

Amount Per Serving

Calories 377.83	Calories from Fat 143

	% DV
Total Fat 15.85g	24%
Cholesterol 39.29mg	13%
Sodium 914.76mg	38%
Total Carbohydrate 44.59g	15%
Protein 14.07g	28%

Unofficial Pts: 9 ©DietFacts.com
(Fiber unknown so Pts may be lower)

Percent of Calories from:
Fat: 37.8% Carb: 47.2% Protein: 14.9%
(Total may not equate 100% due to rounding.)

*Percent Daily Values (DV) are based on a 2,000 calorie diet. Your daily values may be higher or lower depending on your calorie needs:

Nutrient		2,000 Calories	2,500 Calories
Total Fat	less than	65 g	80 g
Saturated Fat	less than	20 g	25 g
Cholesterol	less than	300 mg	300 mg
Sodium	less than	2400 mg	2400 mg
Total Carbohydrates		300 g	375 g
Fiber		25 g	30 g

1 g Fat = 9 calories 1 g Carbohydrate = 4 calories
1 g Protein = 4 calories 1 g Alcohol = 7 calories

Source: dietfacts.com

Why Do We Eat?

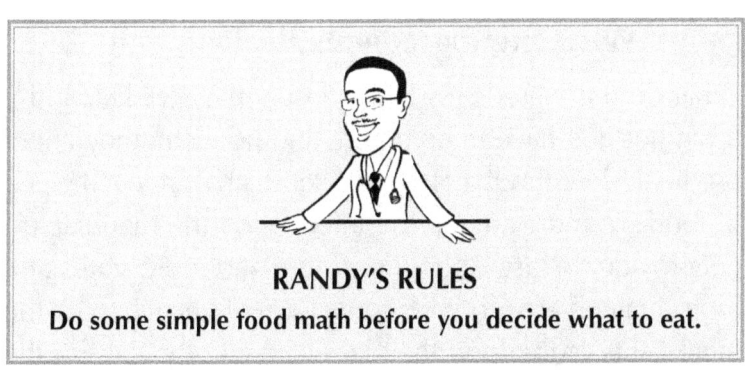

RANDY'S RULES
Do some simple food math before you decide what to eat.

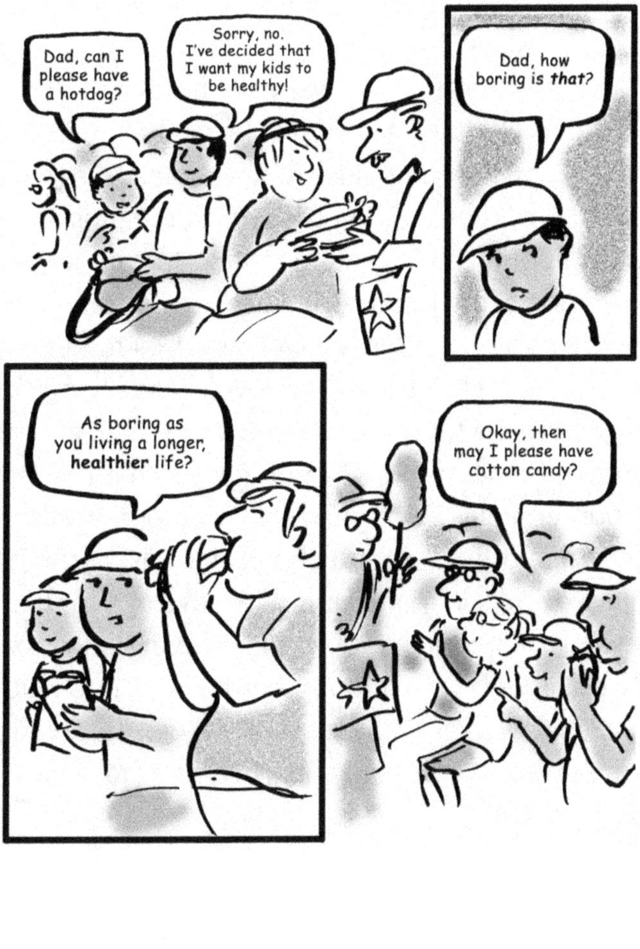

What the Ingredients Really Mean

What do the ingredients in a Whopper, a Twinkie, and a basic hot dog have in common, and how can they affect our health? Without a chemistry kit to analyze each piece of food we must rely on the information the manufacturers provide. In fast-food joints, more and more states and municipalities are requiring some form of signage to list the ingredients of the food they are selling. In the case of the generic hot dog, we can do some simple research online to discover its make-up.

What are these labels really telling us? The Percent Daily Value (% DV) is supposed to be a guide to the nutrients in one serving of food, since it tells the percentage of that nutrient that you should be eating—if you were to eat only that one item in a 2000 calorie diet on any given day. The Food and Drug Administration (FDA) recommends Percent Daily Value as a tool to determine whether or not a food is high or low in specific nutrients. For example, if a food has 5 percent or less of a particular nutrient it's considered to be low in that nutrient. If that food contains 20 percent or more of that nutrient, it's considered high. Sound confusing? It is. Many of us, concerned with our daily fat intake, have trouble figuring out exactly how much fat we might be ingesting, based solely on label information. According to Anne Dubner, our resident dietician, there's a quick way to determine how much fat is really in a particular food when you examine its label.

"I call it the 'Dubner Handy Fat Calculator,'" she says. "Round off the calories per serving and divide that number by 50. That's how many grams of fat make up 20 percent of your calories. This is less than the American Heart Association recommends, but it's good to aim low in case you have a bit more."

Anne goes on to describe her easy method for determining fat content.

"Let's look at the food label for that hot dog. It has a whopping 378 calories! If you round that number off to the nearest 50, that would be 400. Now, divide 400 by 50 and you get eight. That's how many grams of fat you *want* to see on that label. But oh my goodness! This hot dog has 16 grams of fat! That's double what you want—40 percent of calories from fat."

And, what about sodium, another one of the big, bad three: sugar, salt, and fat? Look at the calories per serving and the milligram count of sodium. It should not be more than two times the calories. The hot dog would be heart healthy if it had about 750 mg of sodium. Unfortunately, it has 915! And that's just in one dog! How many of you can eat just one? What about the bun? And the ketchup? And the chips or French fries you might be eating along with it?

Love of Self, Family, and Community

Utilizing everything we have discussed so far, we can now begin to realign ourselves with the spiritual mission of becoming healthy—as a means for loving ourselves, our families, our friends, and our communities in a deeper, more comprehensive way. When we look at health from this perspective, it clearly becomes much more than a matter of losing weight, buying the right kind of food, and doing push-ups. When we accept the fact that corporate greed may always trump morality, we can simply focus on personal responsibility and instilling a quality set of values for our entire family. It's not just something to be addressed in the privacy of our homes. It should be a subject brought to the forefront of each and every community in our country.

In the world of organized religion I would like to see preachers, imams, and rabbis challenging their followers to become healthier. I would like to hear them asking their congregations, at each and every service, these questions:

1. How many of you walked here today?
2. How many of you have cars outside, right now, in the parking lot? Of course, we understand that some people have good reasons for not walking. But what about the rest of you, who live close enough to walk?
3. How much money are you wasting today, driving a short distance from your home to get here, just because it's convenient?
4. How many of you took a minute to consider what effect your car has had on your environment?

Why Do We Eat?

5. How many of you wondered what it could be like to enjoy a leisurely stroll with your wife or husband and children?

I can hear the priest and the imam and the rabbi cajoling members of their churches, mosques, and synagogues to come together—but on foot, using the bodies the Lord has given them.

Any Western clergy might choose to cite a story from the Old Testament, found in the first book of Daniel, when King Nebuchadnezzar, the king of Babylon, decreed that certain children he had captured from the tribes of Israel should be prepared to enter the king's service. But first, over a three-year period, they were all to be fed the food and drink of the king, himself. Daniel, inspired by his spiritual leanings, insisted on not defiling himself with a heavy diet of meat and wine. Instead, he managed to convince the king's eunuch to let him eat vegetables and drink water for a ten-day trial period, after which all the children would be tested to see who fared best. Not surprisingly, Daniel was deemed to be the healthiest of everyone and he eventually had great influence in the king's court.

Each of us can be Daniel, exercising self-control for the good of our own health as well as positively influencing those around us, even those in positions of authority. And it can start quite nicely, right at home. Imagine your son or daughter, sitting at the dinner table, turning down the spare ribs you're about to offer and asking for stir-fry vegetables and brown rice instead. Imagine your husband rejecting soda, drinking water, and replacing cake with a piece of fresh fruit for dessert. With the proper education and encouragement, these things could happen right in your very own home. It starts with you. Are you ready to accept the responsibility?

STOP!

EXERCISE BREAK!

I hope this discussion of fast food has not reminded you to go get some!

If so, have some self-control. Instead of making such a bad choice, do your 10 minutes (minimum) of exercise and then keep reading!

10 minutes! Three times a day (at least). You can do it. You *should* do it.

Your life depends on it! Think of all the people depending on you.

If you're too stubborn to get healthy for yourself, at least do it for them!

Ten minutes. Right now. Come on. Take it slow.

Put on some music. Get moving and enjoy yourself. Get HEALTHY!

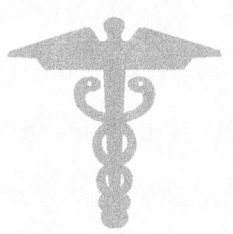

The Wright Reminders

Ask yourself why you eat.

Choose foods wisely.

Investigate ingredients.

Do the math.

Exercise!

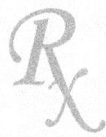

CHAPTER 5

Are You Really Smarter Than Your Doctor?

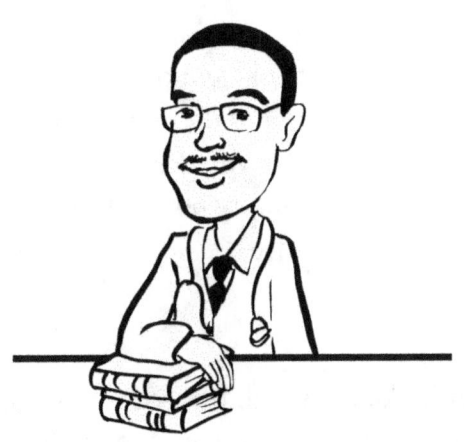

Oops—More Denial

We are a nation obsessed with outward appearances and all too often we ignore what's going on inside of ourselves, both physically and spiritually. Many diseases, which afflict far too many people, could be avoided by paying much keener attention to what we eat, how we exercise, and how much love we allow in our lives.

> **STOP!**
>
> **EXERCISE BREAK!**
>
> Here we go again. Get moving!
>
> So glad I mentioned it.
>
> Once again:
> Put down the book, turn on some music, and do your favorite 10 minutes!
>
> And watch what you drink afterward.
> Avoid the sugary power drinks.
>
> Try water.

Rather than looking inward, our society is obsessed with fixing things externally. Madison Avenue tells us that we should be thinner, stronger, smarter, faster, and sexier. They promise a host of products that promise to provide us with all those benefits. Many people literally buy into their messages and spend a fortune each year on a vast array of products, ranging from diet plans to specialized running shoes, from spa cures to new and improved vitamin and miracle supplements (more on that in Chapter 10).

As a society, we also operate on a daily basis in great denial, largely ignoring what can go wrong with our bodies because we have such a bountiful display of supposed solutions and wonder cures at our disposal. It's so much easier to buy a product at the store or order it online than to actually call our doctor, make an appointment, and go see him or her to discuss our situation. Entertaining any notion that something could be wrong with our health causes us great dis–ease. The thought of being sick, let alone facing a life-threatening illness, can simply ruin what looked like an ordinary day. But the truth is, whether we want to face it or not, too many people are living dangerously and flirting with disaster.

Once you understand how diseases happen, you might be able to avoid them, not just for yourself but for your family members as well.

The Curse of Childhood Obesity

Obese: (adjective) extremely and unhealthily fat

According to the Centers for Disease Control and Prevention, one third of America's youth is now overweight and at serious risk for developing high blood pressure, high cholesterol, and diabetes. Many are stigmatized and bullied by their peers and teachers, and suffer from low self-esteem, which can lead to depression, compromised academic achievement, and diminished life quality.

The American Diabetes Association predicts that nearly one out of three kids born in 2000 (and one in two minorities) will develop type 2 diabetes in his or her lifetime.

Obese children are more than twice as likely to die prematurely as adults than kids on the lower end of the weight spectrum. The World Health Organization is calling it a crisis of "epidemic proportions."

Does any of this ring a bell? Do you recognize anyone in your family, school, or neighborhood who you would honestly consider obese? Chances are you do because America now leads the developing world in its rate of obesity. The annual negative cost of obesity (for medical treatment, lost hours of productivity, etc.) is now pushing $150 billion! The National Institute of Diabetes and Digestive and Kidney Diseases states that "Obesity means having too much body fat. It is different from being overweight, which means weighing too much. The weight may come from muscle, bone, fat and/or body water.

Both terms—obese and overweight—mean that a person's weight is greater than what's considered healthy for his or her height. Obesity occurs over time when you eat more calories than you use. The balance between calories-in and calories-out differs for each person. Factors that might tip the balance include your genetic makeup, overeating, eating high-fat foods, and not being physically active. If you are obese, losing even 5 to 10 percent of your weight can delay or prevent problems such as heart disease, stroke, arthritis, and some cancers.

The White House Task Force on Childhood Obesity, founded in 2010 by First Lady Michelle Obama, is dedicated to tackling the challenge of what some call a national plague. Most of their recommendations are targeted at institutions outside of the home; for example, improving the food supply in America's public schools, as well as working with the food and beverage industry to limit the marketing of unhealthy products, especially for children. They are also encouraging schools to bring back daily physical education classes and increase the amount of recess time for elementary school children.

While each of these campaigns is indisputably valuable, as with any type of educational and behavioral shift for children, it must begin at home! With you, the parents and guardians of our children. We all know that the food and beverage industry will go only as far as its profit margins permit. With public schools struggling to stay open and prosper, spending any additional monies on physical education equipment may not be a priority. Sadly, it's the children who lose.

The responsibility for our children's long-term health prognosis lies with the adults at home who are their primary caretakers. Parents, grandparents, extended family members, and professional nannies must take it upon themselves to learn how to do this. Whether it means acquiring the necessary knowledge, encouraging behavioral changes, laying down the law, or any combination of the three, something must be done immediately.

Whatever pediatricians, teachers, and parents have been doing up until now is obviously not working. Statistics prove it. Just open your eyes and look around. You will notice that there are way too many people carrying around way too much weight, and way too many of them are children. One of them might be yours.

But they didn't end up this way by themselves. It's not their fault. These kids are minors. They are our responsibility! We must take charge of their lives and ensure them some modicum of a healthy future.

Albert Einstein defined insanity as doing the same thing over and over again and expecting different results. With this definition in mind, the way we have been treating childhood obesity qualifies as insanity.

Do the math. If you eat more calories than you burn off, you gain weight. There's no avoiding that fact, no matter how much you might try. No amount of rationalization will change the consequences of human science. Eat too much and exercise too little, you gain weight. Keep that combination up and you get fat. Get too fat and you get sick. Get too sick and you die. You can't cheat science!

But it doesn't have to be this way. We, as parents, educators, and citizens, can stop the madness. The first place to start is in our own homes with our own families. We can control our own well-being. There are also plenty of organizations devoted to reducing childhood obesity and getting America's children fit and healthy. They are available to provide all kinds of help and support. Following are just a few of them.

> **COMBATING OBESITY**
>
> First Lady Michelle Obama is working tirelessly to achieve her goal of significantly reducing childhood obesity in America during the course of the next generation.
> For more information, please visit
> **www.letsmove.gov**
>
> *
>
> The National Football League is committed to challenging America's kids to exercise every day for at least 60 minutes.
> Please visit the website at
> **www.nflrush.com/play60**
>
> *
>
> MeMe Roth, the founder and president of National Action Against Obesity, encourages everyone to lend a hand in fighting against childhood obesity.
>
> "Let's finally recognize obesity as abuse—abuse of our children, abuse of ourselves—and together take action against it."
> **www.actionagainstobesity.com**
>
> *
>
> The Recipe for Success Foundation was launched in 2005 by Gracie and Bob Cavnar to lead the way in hands-on nutrition education, aimed at preventing childhood obesity and encouraging long term health.
> **www.recipe4success.org**

Me, Me, Me!!!

We all have egos, which can motivate us, act as protection, or simply get in our way as developing human beings. The

"I" syndrome, this self-centeredness we all maintain, is both unhealthy and surprisingly dangerous, especially when it comes to our health.

"I am fine."

"I am not overweight."

"I will change my habits tomorrow."

"I can't exercise. I don't have time."

"I don't have money to join a gym."

I. I. I. Look at all the attention we place on ourselves with nothing to show for it, except perhaps a steadily inflating body, a compromised spirit, and a host of developing health issues.

None of this, unfortunately, is limited to children.

"Obesity now accounts for 10 percent of the healthcare costs in the U.S. and $147 billion, and smoking accounts for $100 billion," says Delos M. Cosgrove, MD, CEO and

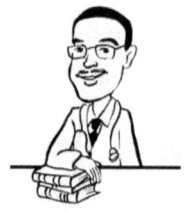

THE WRIGHT ADVICE

Poor nutrition is linked to low disease resistance, lack of energy, heart diseases, and cancer. Poor nutrition is not always related to economics. It can be simply a result of bad choices. You have the opportunity to decide.

Don't you want to increase your chances of being healthy?

president of the Cleveland Clinic. "We could provide a lot of healthcare if we didn't have those two big problems."

The Teenager Syndrome

Life is great as a teenager. I can recall my high school years when my idols were Ferris Bueller and Marty McFly. I spent many nights watching *Star Trek* reruns and speculating with friends about whether George Lucas would make any sequels. It was a time of innocence and invincibility. It was a time when I was more worried about the here and now, and I had faith that the future would take care of itself. As with most teenagers, I embraced adulthood with a vague sense of excitement, but was not really clear how to get there. My parents told me what I needed to do, but their redundant instructions often fell on unreceptive ears. I knew they were right, but the future seemed so far away that I could not see how their message had any practical, real-world application.

Many of us treat our health like a teenager treats his future. I call this the Teenager Syndrome. We know that taking care of ourselves is important. We know that certain foods are bad for us. We know we should not drink or smoke excessively, but the effect of such behaviors takes so long to develop that many people feel that any single action done today isn't really going to matter next week. Well, just like getting a C on a single ninth grade algebra test is not going to be the main reason a teenager doesn't become the CEO of a Fortune 500 company, a series of poor grades in several key classes may.

The same is true with our health. While occasional indulgences will most likely not alter our ultimate state of health, a lifestyle of indulgences certainly will catch up to us and eventually wreak havoc. In a society centered around convenience, easy living, and a "right now" mentality, it is easy to see how the temptation to indulge on a regular basis can easily break down most people's defenses.

Like with most teenagers who eventually "saw the light" and began to live their lives along the straight and narrow, it typically takes an "aha" moment for many of us to realize that we need to start living right. In my experience, many people behave in a way described by country music star Tim McGraw, in his song "Live Like You Were Dying." They wait until a tragic, near-death experience occurs before taking their lives seriously. Like the man in the song, do you really want to wait until you're in your early 40s before you start living a healthier life? If you can't imagine it for yourself, how about for those who love you and need you?

The good news is we don't have to wait until we are near death before changing our lives for the better. This book can help you adopt a healthy lifestyle now, before it's too late. Study after study suggests that our actions today can directly affect our future health. In this chapter, we shall learn about several major health conditions that are potentially life threatening, but through proper action, may be preventable.

I hope you never get to know these diseases firsthand, or through a loved one or friend, but perhaps knowing about them will inspire you to live a life that ultimately discourages any of them from ever entering your life.

Disease States Revealed

Any one of a handful of major diseases, be it an affliction of the heart, the lungs, diabetes, cancer, or stroke, can set the stage for long-term consequences. While any of these diseases (and many others) may take years to develop, they can change a person's life in the blink of an eye. With that in mind, wouldn't it be worth anyone's time to learn more about these potential killers and do whatever possible to avoid developing one of them? You do have a choice! Although genetics does play an indisputable role in our health, the threat of a stroke, heart disease, lung disease, diabetes, and even cancer can be averted by living a conscientious, healthy, and mindful lifestyle.

Stroke

As a child, I often played with my grandfather. I loved how he threw me up in the air and caught me just before I hit the ground. I loved hearing his stories of World War II, because he was a heroic sergeant in the Army. My grandfather was a great soldier and survived many difficult battles. However, the most devastating blow he ever encountered occurred right inside his very own home!

In a single day, my grandfather went from being a strong, jovial, energetic person to someone who could not speak or walk, and needed my grandmother's help just to use the bathroom. He certainly couldn't throw me up in the air anymore.

At the time, I didn't understand what had happened. No one really explained to me why my grandfather was so suddenly different. I knew only that PaPa was sick, and we had to be quiet in the house so he could rest. It wasn't until years later, when I was in medical school, that I finally understood what had happened to my grandfather. He'd had a stroke!

Maybe my PaPa left me with a special mission to fight the war against heart disease and stroke. That could be why I direct two stroke centers and spend so much of my time spreading the message of risk-factor modification. Maybe it is destiny that you are reading this book, because it may actually save your life if you learn even one of the lessons being taught.

"Stroke ain't no joke."

Well, it isn't. It is a devastating condition that's the leading cause of disability in North America. According to a 2010 CDC report, stroke is now the fourth leading cause of death, after heart disease, cancer, and respiratory ailments. The American Heart Association has embarked on a major campaign to educate people, including doctors, about the dangers of stroke. With the advent of more stroke centers, increased use of clot busting drugs, and people reading books like this, I am encouraged that we can fight this disease. The principles discussed in this chapter (and others) may conceivably save your life or the life of a loved one or friend.

What causes a stroke? A stroke occurs when there is a blocked blood vessel in the brain. When this happens, when blood and oxygen stop flowing, the brain begins to die.

Blood pressure is a measure of the pressure inside those tiny blood vessels. As the systolic blood pressure rises above 120 (the top number), the pressure is great enough to actually create small tears in the lining of the blood vessel, typically near sharp bends in the vessel. These tears serve as entry points for fat cells that tend to narrow a blood vessel. To add insult to injury, just like a blood clot forms on your skin when you cut yourself, a blood clot forms at the site of a tearing in the lining of a blood vessel.

When this happens in a constricting area, the blood vessel narrows even more and can block off completely! If the blood vessel goes to the brain it forces a stroke. If the blood vessel goes to the heart, it creates a heart attack. In either case, it can be devastating.

The more fatty foods you eat and the higher your blood pressure, the more at risk you are for a stroke or heart attack. Diabetes, which we will discuss momentarily, serves as an accelerator for this process by speeding up the narrowing of the arteries.

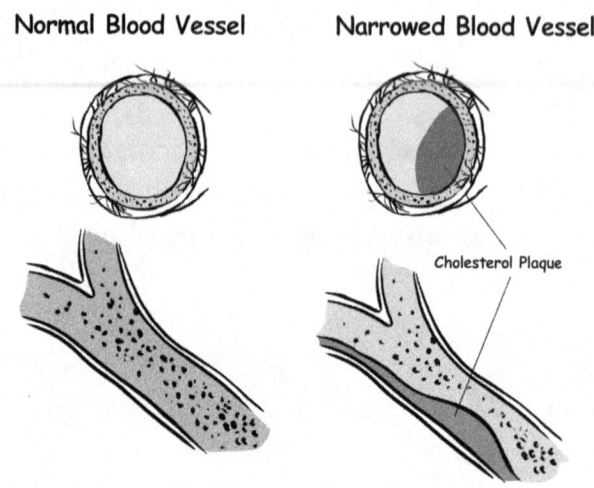

The Brain

The brain is an amazing organ with millions of functions. It is the source of our thoughts, memories, and desires, as well as the host of our five senses.

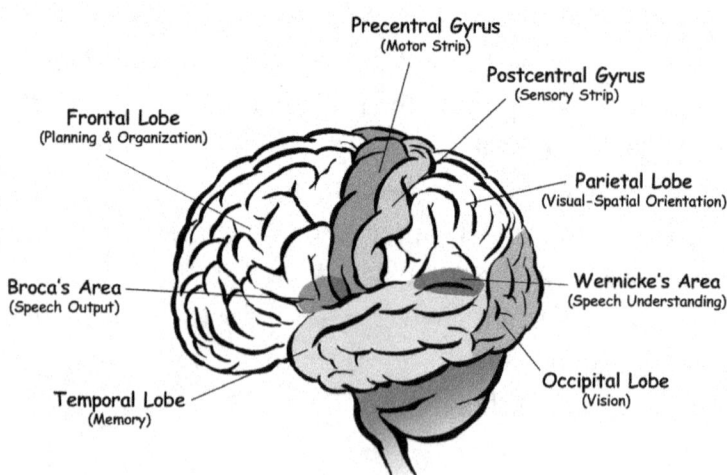

There is essentially no function that we perform on a daily basis that our brain doesn't control. Because of this, the symptoms from a stroke can vary, as they are directly related to the specific part of the brain that becomes deprived of oxygen by the blocked artery. Most people do not even recognize the signs and symptoms of a stroke. When that happens, the consequences can be terribly serious, if not fatal.

Common Signs of a Stroke

Sudden onset of numbness and/or weakness on one side of the body

Difficulty speaking

Sudden visual loss

Sudden difficulty with balance and walking

New and severe headache

If you experience any of these symptoms, consider it an emergency and call 911 immediately. Every second you waste debating whether you should or should not go to the hospital means the literal possibility of your brain cells dying. Most of us can't afford to lose any more brain cells, so don't waste any time if you think you are at risk.

GET TO THE EMERGENCY ROOM IMMEDIATELY!

Time loss = brain loss.

Heart Disease

The American Heart Association does a great job of getting its message to millions of people around the world. Instead of repeating its advice, I'd like to remind you about the risk factors associated with heart attacks. Technically speaking, a heart attack occurs when blood flow to the heart via the coronary arteries is blocked. When a heart attack occurs, the heart muscle is damaged and can no longer pump blood properly. This effectively makes the heart a much less efficient pump and puts you at risk for heart failure down the line.

The same relationship between high blood pressure, diabetes, and high cholesterol that we discussed earlier in the Stroke section holds true here as well. Having any of these three risk factors can dramatically increase one's chances of developing a heart attack or stroke (so just imagine your chances if you have two or even all three of these factors).

Smoking and excessive alcohol use are the two changeable risk factors (even though I also consider physical inactivity and unhealthy eating to be changeable risk factors). So minimizing your risk factors will decrease your chance for developing a heart attack.

Straight from the Heart

Heart attacks, like strokes, are preventable! Know your risk factors, change those you can control, and recognize the warning signs, which include:

1. Chest discomfort. It may be a sharp pain, a tightness, pressure, or squeezing, or it has even

been described as an elephant sitting on your chest.
2. Discomfort in the upper body, including the jaw, back, arms or stomach.
3. Shortness of breath.
4. Related symptoms include nausea, sweating, and lightheadedness.
5. Women sometimes experience the related symptoms and NOT the typical chest pain. So ladies, please pay extra attention for any atypical sensations you may experience and keep a low threshold for getting yourself evaluated.

Diabetes

According to Me

I've always been in good health. I never went to a doctor until my wife, aka "Dr. Mom," noticed I was going to the bathroom more than usual. She also noticed me complaining about feeling worn-out and tired. She basically dragged me to the doctor to get tested. Lab work revealed that my glucose was high. The doctor diagnosed me with diabetes and put me on a strict diet. Luckily, we caught it early. With encouragement from my wife, I maintain close to normal glucose levels with two pills a day, a new diet, and daily exercise. My only complication has been a little numbness in my feet, but it hasn't progressed in the five years I have been under a doctor's care.

Melvin, age 65, Hartford, Connecticut

"DocSpeak"

Melvin is blessed to have an observant wife, who noticed his symptoms and made him take action. She did what more people should do. She paid attention and spoke up! With his doctor's guidance and compliance with the prescribed comprehensive treatment plan, Melvin should do quite well.

Diabetes is a condition that results in the body's abnormal handling of glucose. People who are not able to control their diabetes face any number of complications when high blood glucose persists over a long period of time. It can lead to blindness and other visual problems. In the feet, the high blood sugar can damage the nerves, resulting in what we call a neuropathy. The damage to the nerves initially results in a burning sensation, or numbness in the feet, and can eventually lead to a complete loss of sensation. This can be dangerous because people can injure or cut themselves and not even know it. Because diabetics heal slower than non-diabetics, small cuts can result in large, non-healing ulcers, which may eventually need amputation if medical attention is not sought early.

Three Types of Diabetes

Type 1:
This form is typically diagnosed in children and young adults. It used to be called juvenile diabetes, and it affects 5 to 10 percent of the population. It results from the body not producing any insulin at all! Insulin is a hormone made by the body that removes glucose from the blood and moves

it into various cells in the body, where the glucose is to be used a fuel source. This results in a buildup of glucose in the blood, which over time can damage other organs. Individuals with this type of diabetes are usually on insulin therapy, which typically involves taking insulin shots on a daily basis.

Type 2:
This is the most common form, and is often called adult-onset diabetes. It affects millions of Americans, and many are not even aware they have it. Type 2 diabetes occurs when the body is either not producing enough insulin or the cells in the body are not responding properly to insulin. Either way, glucose is not moving correctly from the bloodstream into the cells, where it's needed. This results in the buildup of glucose in the blood stream, which can lead to a variety of complications that can affect, for example, your eyes, nerves, kidneys, heart, and skin.

Gestational:
This form affects women who are pregnant, usually starting around 28 weeks. It is typically managed with the help of your doctor, and it does not mean you will have diabetes after delivery, nor does it mean you had it before you became pregnant. It typically results from hormonal imbalances and usually resolves after delivery. It affects about 4 percent of pregnant women.

Other complications resulting from diabetes include high blood pressure, kidney disease, stroke, heart attack, and slow gastric emptying (gastroparesis). Diabetes affects multiple organs and can be a very damaging disease. The good news is that diabetes is very controllable. But it takes discipline and a willingness to make certain lifestyle changes, many of which are outlined in this book.

Obesity is another condition that tends to worsen the effects of diabetes. The exercise and fitness suggestions in Chapter 14 of this book can help improve glucose control. Studies have shown that exercise can significantly reduce blood glucose levels. Diet also plays an important role. Although this book is not designed to serve specifically as a diabetic eating plan, many of the principles introduced here will fit in well with most recommendations provided by the American Diabetic Association. For more specific information about eating and lifestyle changes, speak to your doctor or a dietitian.

Cancer

As we mentioned earlier, cancer, despite its bad reputation, is not the leading cause of death in America. We should be more afraid of getting heart disease than cancer. But most of us fear cancer more because we don't understand how we get it in the first place.

Cancer represents a problem with our cells. Each of the cells in our body has a set time to grow, remain stable, and die. In a perfectly functioning body, each cell performs its job without mistakes. However, one small problem in a cell can change its instructions, and it may start reproducing at a time when it's not supposed to.

This is the essence of a cancer, a set of cells no longer obeying their natural cues, and multiplying out of control. If these cells are in the colon, it is called colon cancer. If the cells are in the breast, it's called breast cancer, and if they are in the prostate, it's called prostate cancer. A tumor is simply a large group of these uncontrolled cells that form a mass, or tumor.

The reason cells get out of control is complicated and depends on the cell types. Each cell in the body (heart, brain, kidney, breast, etc.) has different controls to follow, different responses to change in the environment, and even different genetic makeup. Therefore, finding the exact cause of what makes a cell go from normal reproduction to uncontrolled reproduction is a daunting task. This change is called a mutation and typically occurs in a cell's DNA. Possible causes of mutations include exposures such as chemicals (like asbestos), radiation, excessive sunlight (watch out sun tanners), and, you guessed it—smoking.

Our bodies have natural defenses against such rogue cells. When a cell starts to behave irregularly, it is typically destroyed and removed from the body. However, with cancerous cells, the body is not able to contain the growth of the mutation, and as a result, cancer develops. This process can take years to occur and doesn't always cause any symptoms until the cancer has grown or has spread to other parts of the body.

Most people believe that cancer just happens out of the blue, and in many cases, we still do not understand what "causes" most cancers. However, we now know that certain risk factors exist that may increase one's chances of developing cancer. To me, that's exciting news, because now I may be able to alter my future for the better by doing certain things today.

> ### According to Me
>
> In August 2002, I was limping around with a sore and swollen toe. At night, I would tell my wife that the sheets were too heavy as they lay on my sore toe. Aside from the swelling that would come and go, I felt fine, so we weren't too concerned. I have my own paint and wallpaper business and I thought a spider, while working at a dirty job site, had bitten me.
>
> In September, my hand swelled so much my wedding ring had to be cut off in the emergency room. This swelling would come and go and I was tired a lot, but I thought I was just working too hard. My wife, Donna, thought maybe I had gout, a form of arthritis causing redness, stiffness, and painful swelling in the joints.
>
> In January, my jaw and neck became badly swollen. My dentist recommended I see a doctor, but since I was never sick I didn't even have one. He made an appointment for me with a friend of his for the next day.
>
> When the doctor ordered a battery of tests, we were a little concerned. When he told us he thought it was lymphoma and would be referring me to an oncologist, I was shocked. We never had thought my symptoms meant anything like that.
>
> "But I feel fine," I said. "How could I have cancer?"
>
> *Jim, age 61, Edmond, Oklahoma*

"DocSpeak"

We'll never know if Jim's lifestyle played a significant role in the onset of his initial symptoms, but we can be pretty sure that when Jim began ignoring his symptoms in the summer of 2002 he was setting himself up for some major health consequences.

The simple lesson is that we should never ignore unusual symptoms, in this case a persistently swollen toe, because they often mean something else is going wrong with our bodies. If we catch the problems early enough we may be able to avoid the dire consequences Jim ended up facing with his cancer treatments.

The American Institute for Cancer Research (AICR) has made specific recommendation for all Americans to follow to help reduce their risk of developing cancer. The team that developed these recommendations reviewed all the available data on a variety of cancers, including the relationships between diet, exercise, and weight in regard to cancer prevention.

Prevention

How can we prevent cancer? People are always asking me that. They also want to know how they can fight cancer naturally. I tell them all to buy fruits and veggies and eat them every day. That's it! You don't need fancy herbs flown in from some exotic country, costing you an arm and a leg. You don't need any miracle supplements you see advertised on late-night television. You simply need to increase your daily intake of fruits and vegetables (the real fruits, not the juices) and decrease your addiction to red meat.

Why? Well, there is a large body of legitimate scientific studies that show that minerals, vitamins (not the pills but those found in food), and photochemical derived directly from plants have anti-cancer properties. In addition to their anti-cancer properties, they are also low-calorie alternatives that will help you keep your weight down, which is also a good way to help decrease your chances of getting cancer.

The New American Plate

The results of the AICR's findings are included in an amazing document called the New American Plate, which you can access at www.aicr.org.

The message is simple: In order to reduce the risk of developing cancer, you should eat more plants, less red meat and processed meat, exercise at least 30 minutes a day, maintain a healthy weight, and do not smoke or chew tobacco.

(Please see Chapters 12 and 13 for more extensive information.)

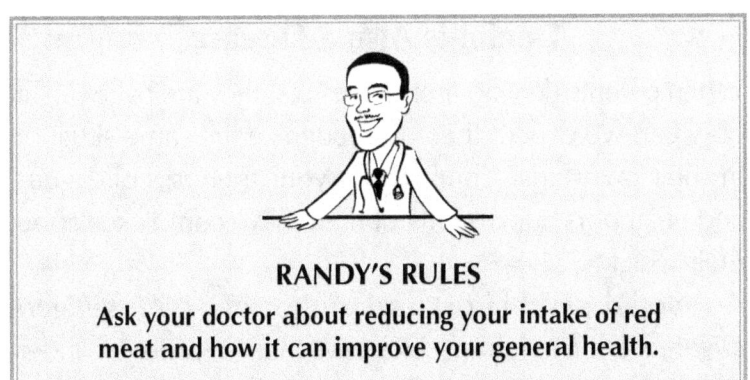

RANDY'S RULES
Ask your doctor about reducing your intake of red meat and how it can improve your general health.

Respiratory Disease

Smoking puts one at high risk for lung cancer and any number of other illnesses and diseases, ranging from the common cold to a fatal bout of pneumonia. The most common respiratory diseases include asthma, chronic bronchitis, emphysema, pulmonary disease and fibrosis, and acidosis. But lung disease can be caused by any number of environmental factors, such as air pollution, asbestos, and other toxic chemicals.

I wonder though if everyone stopped smoking, would respiratory disease still be ranked third on the CDC list of deadly diseases?

Of course it's unrealistic to expect the world to be smoke-free, but if you know smoking can kill you, why not make your best effort to stop?

Denial Is Also a Disease

When parents deny to themselves that they are overweight, how can we expect them to recognize the same situation in their own kids? Think about your friends, colleagues, and neighbors. How many of them have complexes about their weight?

Noted psychiatrist and author of *The Intelligent Divorce,* Dr. Mark Banschick says that "in order to understand complexes, we must return to the topic of denial—the wish not to see what is really there. Complexes have their source in childhood. They go back to early memories of your father, mother, siblings, uncles, aunts, and kids in the community. Mistreatment forms the heart of a complex. Maybe you were criticized, ridiculed, hit, violated, or simply unloved."

Most of us prefer to forget our childhood hurts because remembering too much of them can be overwhelming. But denial can also protect us from pain—to a point. Somewhere along the way, we have to deal with whatever has hurt us. Otherwise, we are left with psychological wounds that, under the right circumstances, can be activated. Human nature teaches us that psychological and emotional trouble often leads to bad personal habits, such as unhealthy eating, drinking, and a major lack of exercise.

We're right back where we started—facing disease. You can avoid a great deal of it if you face up to any patterns of denial you might be exhibiting. Granted, this kind of honesty might be difficult to pull off all alone. Consulting with your doctor or another trained professional might help guide you in the right direction.

But I'm Tired!

Has all this talk of disease made you tired? Not surprising. Stress is exhausting, all by itself, and denial doesn't exactly energize anyone in the long run either. So, for any number of reasons—a lousy diet, lack of exercise, communication issues—we can be stressing ourselves and sleeping poorly. Once we don't sleep well, we kick a vicious cycle into motion.

That brings us to our final topic for this chapter: the issue of sleep and our struggle to get enough good quality shut-eye.

The Struggle for Sleep

As I sit here typing, I look over and see one of my sons sitting up next to me, keeping me company. However, as time passes and I type on, I see his little eyes start to slowly close. They appear to get heavier and heavier with each minute. He fights valiantly to say awake, but the powerful, unrelenting forces of sleep soon overtake him. Why is life so ironic? Normally, my two sons run from sleep, because it's something that interferes with the things they are determined to see and do throughout their busy days. On the other hand, many of us are on a hunt for sleep, and it's nowhere to be found. We try everything we can, but we just can't get the sleep we desire.

As a neurologist who is board certified in sleep medicine, I have the opportunity to work with thousands of individuals with a wide variety of sleep problems. Sleep is a fascinating field, and because it is a state of being that is still not completely understood, it almost feels like we're working on some mysterious edge of humanity.

The reasons why we sleep are still not fully understood. Several theories abound, from energy conservation in times of scant resources (food, water, etc.) to neurocognitive theories that suggest our brains (and bodies) rebuild depleted resources, consolidate memories, and effectively reboots themselves for the next day. Of course our bodies do not technically shut down each night when we sleep, but sleep does seem to serve a similar function to restarting your computer.

As a neurologist, I like the brain-related theories. But despite science's inability to provide a definite answer as to why we sleep, we do know that if we don't, a lot of bad things can happen, and we will eventually die. So, in the interest of prolonging life, let's discuss why we need to sleep, and a few tips on how to get more of it.

Most people need six to eight hour of sleep per day. Sleep can be broken down into two main categories: REM sleep and non-REM sleep. REM (Rapid Eye Movement) sleep is the stage when our brains are extremely active with our brain-wave recordings almost indistinguishable from when we are awake. It is typically very easy to wake someone up during this phase, and most of us dream during this time. One really interesting phenomenon that occurs during this stage is that our muscles are paralyzed. It's often believed that this occurs so that we do not act out our dreams.

Brain activity slows down during non-REM sleep. Its stages are numbered one to four, with one being the lightest and four the deepest. It is hard to wake some one out of Stage Four sleep. Believe me, when my sons are in that state, you can take them out of bed, change their diaper, and return them to bed without them ever knowing. Throughout a typical night, our body will cycle through about four 90-minute cycles. The cycles include Stages One to Four, then a REM cycle, then possibly a brief arousal, and then it starts all over again.

When you are not sleeping well, the need to sleep presents itself as a feeling of chronic tiredness. This is typically accompanied by a rise of adenosine in your body (and guess what, caffeine blocks adenosine, thus making you feel less sleepy).

Many people who complain of excessive daytime sleepiness are found to have either poor sleep hygiene, side effects from medication, another medical problem that disturbs their sleep (like needing to go to the bathroom frequently at night), or poor sleep due to pain. Others may have an underlying sleep problem like obstructive sleep apnea, narcolepsy, or even primary hypersomnolence. All these condition produce excessive daytime sleepiness, and if you have any of these symptoms, you should see your doctor.

Insomnia is a condition the affects people all over the world. Its causes are varied. In my practice, before I start anyone on medication to help induce sleep, I put them on a proper sleep schedule. Children are not the only ones who benefit from a routine sleep schedule! The adult brain functions best when it has a predictable schedule to follow in regard to sleep. People who do not subscribe to a consistent schedule of sleeping and waking are likely to eventually develop some form of a sleep complaint. So, if the time you fall asleep at night is based upon the boredom you feel because nothing good is on one of those 340 channels, watch out: you may end up in my office sooner than you think.

How to Sleep

1. **Get the bedroom cool before you go to bed.** Most people sleep better if their room is dark and cool.
2. **Take a warm bath or shower before you go to bed.** The fall in body temperature signals the brain that it is time to go to sleep.
3. **Drink warm milk or some other noncaffeinated beverage before you go to bed.** Once again, the fall in body temperature from warm back to cool tells the brain it's time to sleep. If you go to the bathroom frequently at night, you should skip this tip.

4. **Develop a pre-sleep routine.** Doing your favorite relaxing activity is a good way to wind down from the day. Listening to calming music or reading are great ways to end your day. Try to avoid stimulating activities.
5. **Do all worrying before going to bed.** This is easier said than done, but you should make a conscious decision to think and reflect on your day *before* you go to your room to sleep. If you can adapt this routine, it can save you many restless nights. But be patient. This takes practice.
6. **Go to your bedroom only when you are sleepy.**
7. **If you cannot sleep after 15 to 20 minutes or you wake up at some point during the night, and cannot fall back to sleep after 15 to 20 minutes, then get out of bed.** Go to a dimly lit section of your home and do a relaxing activity until you feel sleepy again. Once you feel sleepy, return to your bedroom.
8. **Do not exercise before going to bed.** Working out tends to raise the level of excitatory neurotransmitters, and in many people, this can interfere with sleep.
9. **Avoid naps during the day (for adults).**
10. **No caffeine after lunch.** It tends to stay in your system and can interfere with sleep.

11. **No alcohol within six hours of sleep.** Many people feel that alcohol helps them sleep. The reality is that alcohol will put you to sleep pretty quickly. However, as it gets metabolized in the liver over the next several hours, its breakdown products tend to disrupt sleep, and you will soon be uncomfortable and your sleep will be disrupted. So don't fall for the age-old trap of a glass of wine before you go to bed.
12. **Avoid watching TV or other stimulating activity in your bed prior to going to sleep.** In sensitive people, these activities may interfere with falling asleep.

These techniques are widely used to help people improve their sleep hygiene. Getting the proper amount of sleep is critical for us to function at our best. Studies have shown that sleep deprivation has been associated with impaired glucose tolerance; increased blood pressure; abnormalities in appetite, which may contribute to obesity; slow, cognitive activity and memory problems; lapses in attention; and depressed moods.

This list includes but a few of the many ailments that can arise from a chronic lack of sleep. It's important for you to realize that burning the candle on both ends will literally make you lose your candle. Sleep is critical, so make sure you get enough. Before you reach for a sleeping pill, try putting the tips in this chapter to good use.

Improving your nutrition, incorporating fitness, and getting consistently good sleep will give you more energy, a clearer mind, and a healthier body.

For more information on all of these topics, visit our website at www.TheWrightChoiceRx.com.

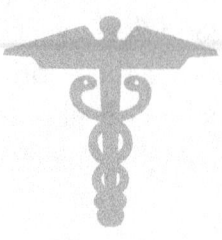

The Wright Reminders

Educate yourself about disease.

Write down all your excuses.

Consult your doctor.

Be honest about denial.

Evaluate your sleeping patterns.

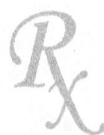

Part Two

Understanding What Makes You Healthy

CHAPTER 6

What Should We Eat? Carbohydrates 101

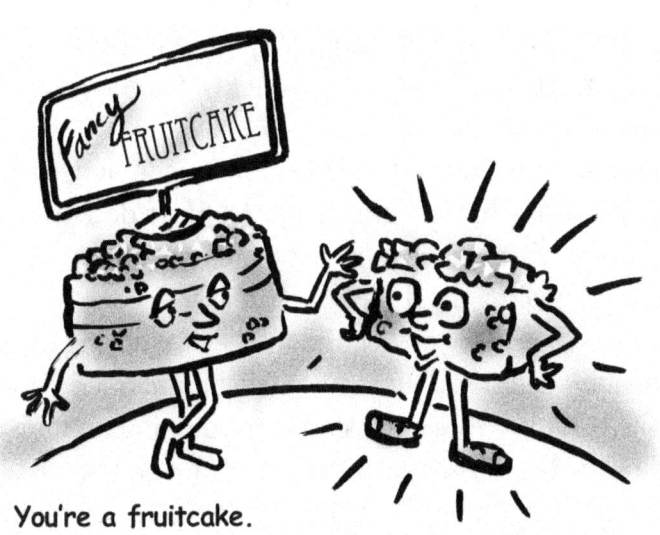

You're a fruitcake.

Yes, but I'm a very *healthy* fruitcake!

Your Energy Handbook

We could write a whole book about the perils of fast food and junk food. But what about the food we eat every day that we consider healthy, or at least not *un*healthy? Advertising assaults us 24/7, at home, on the road, and in the movies, imploring us to eat more and more, claiming, "It's all natural!" Opening up a magazine, a newspaper, or a supermarket circular and trying to make sense of all the information jumping off the page could make anyone dizzy.

Low-carb diets! Low-fat foods! Organically grown fruits and vegetables! Free-range chickens! (Are they really free?) No antibiotics! Locally grown food! Trans fats! Saturated fats! Omega-3 fatty acids! Gluten free! All natural! Aaaahhhhh!!!

It seems like you need a PhD in nutrition to understand anything about what you are eating. All these descriptions can be somewhat intimidating if you are trying to buy food and plan a healthy meal for your family.

But knowledge is power and the key to making effective, healthy decisions. Most everything mentioned above is positive. Most. Your next step is developing an understanding of the basics of nutrition. But don't worry. It doesn't actually require a PhD to figure out the terminology and what it means for you and your family. Over the next few chapters, we will explain many key concepts of nutrition and tie them all together to allow you to better execute and appreciate your decision to live a healthier life. What better place to start than with the food whose primary purpose is to give us energy.

Before we welcome you to the world of carbohydrates I must warn you that this will not be an open invitation to load up on pasta and pizza and other high-carb delights. It's precisely those foods that we need to better understand so that we ingest them properly and in the right amounts and combinations.

Carbohydrates: Friend or Enemy?

We hear a lot about carbohydrates, commonly known as carbs, and the rumors are often negative. You may have noticed friends or family members trying some new version of a low-carb diet in order to lose weight. But do they really understand what they're doing?

Remember my friend who thought he was helping himself by skipping the bun and eating just the hamburger? He didn't really want the meat in the first place, especially a hospital burger. But he, like many others, fell into the carb trap, believing that carbohydrates are the enemy and must be avoided at all cost.

Perhaps the real enemy is hunger, and fighting the urge to satisfy it by any means possible. My friend could've opted to eat any number of other choices offered in the hospital cafeteria. Why didn't he make a more sensible choice? To be honest, he allowed himself to be a creature of habit and a potential victim of taking the path of least resistance.

So the answer to whether carbohydrates are our friend or our enemy is simple. They can be both, depending on the choices we make. You'll discover in this chapter that most of what you probably have heard about carbohydrates has been misleading marketing spins of medical facts. We will show you which carbs are essential to our health and which ones should be avoided.

Simple and Complex—but Simply Sugar

Carbohydrates are a very important part of our daily diet. They are a source of energy-filled nutrients that our bodies need in order to survive and thrive. Carbohydrates are classified as either simple or complex, based on the number of single sugar molecules (monosaccharides) they contain.

You may have heard of the terms glucose, fructose, and galactose, which are three examples of simple sugars.

Glucose is the most well known. It provides energy to our bodies and is the basic building block for all other complex sugars. When we eat carbohydrates, our bodies break them down into glucose to use as energy throughout various parts of our body.

For example, when you eat a sandwich cookie, which is composed of a variety of complex carbohydrates (hard to imagine a simple cookie as "complex"), it starts the digestive process as it enters your mouth. The main area of digestion, however, is in the small intestines. That's where chemicals from your pancreas (called enzymes) break down those complex carbohydrates into simple glucose, fructose, or galactose. The simple sugars then travel to

What Should We Eat? Carbohydrates 101

your liver, where fructose and galactose are ultimately converted into glucose.

Your body doesn't like high levels of glucose in your blood, which is wise, because it can cause a lot of damage, like diabetes. So it fights back by secreting insulin, forcing the glucose back in its cell. Since most of the cells in your body use only what glucose they need, the leftover glucose is stored in your muscles and liver as glycogen, also known as fat! That means if you consume more glucose than your body needs, it ends up as fat. Translation? All those sandwich cookies you may have been eating while reading this book are adding inches to your waistline. (Almost time to exercise, right?)

Your True Blood—aka—the Glycemic Index

Let's not throw away those cookies just yet. As you eat one little treat, your glucose level begins to rise in your bloodstream. The Glycemic Index (GI) measures how fast this happens. The higher the GI, the faster your glucose level rises.

The speed at which your glucose level rises is important because of one thing: insulin. Quickly rising levels of glucose lead to rapidly rising levels of insulin, which try to counter the effects of the glucose. This can result in a drop in your blood sugar level, which makes you crave more simple carbs, also known as "wanting more sweets!" Some scientists believe that people who continuously eat a large proportion of food with a high Glycemic Index are overstimulating their body's production of insulin, which can result in the development of insulin resistance, diabetes, and possibly obesity.

Individuals with diabetes fare better when they plan their meals using the Glycemic Index, ensuring that they keep their blood glucose levels low. If you crave sugary foods, always seem to be thirsty, and have noticed an increase in your need to run to the bathroom, you should see you doctor to be tested for diabetes.

Complex but Not Complicated

Complex carbohydrates (polysaccharides) may sound complicated but they are really not much different than simple carbs. They come in three forms: starch, glycogen, and fiber.

Starch is the storage form of glucose in plants. Plants create glucose by photosynthesis, and the extra glucose is stored in the plant's stems, roots, and seeds in the form of starch. Translation? When we eat a plant or vegetable our bodies convert the starch into glucose, which contains sugar. Humans store extra glucose in the form of glycogen. These glucose stores can be found in our liver and muscles and are called upon to maintain an adequate glucose level in our blood, meaning that sugar in the potato is okay for you, as long as it doesn't become more than your body needs to keep in storage.

Excessive amounts of glycogen are often converted to a more efficient form of storage, commonly known as fat! We will go into this in more detail in Chapter 8, but now you can see how obesity in its simplest form can result from excessive stores of energy, which ultimately comes from what we eat!

Translation? Eating less high-energy food results in less energy available for us to use, which forces our bodies to use its own energy stores, which then starts to deplete our stored energy, which ultimately means we lose fat. Less is less. On the other hand, if we eat a consistent amount of food and increase our body's demand for energy, then we ultimately use more of our stored energy and reduce the amount of fat we are storing. More is more. Translation? Losing weight occurs when we take in less energy than we use!

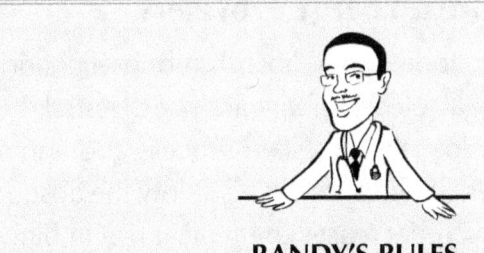

RANDY'S RULES
Avoid unnecessary, excessive amounts of sugar.
Maximize your intake of whole grains, fruits, and veggies.
Eat the skin of the fruit, where the fiber is located!

Fiber

The final complex carbohydrate worth mentioning is fiber. Fiber is a mixture of plant cell-wall material that our bodies are not able to digest. This may sound useless, but it is not.

Fiber is important to help clear our digestive track and add bulk to our stool. The best source of fiber is whole grains.

There are some soluble forms of fiber, which dissolve in water, and they include beans, oats, some vegetables, most fruits, and whole grains. It is the soluble fibers that are helpful in lowering our cholesterol levels and improving glucose control in people with diabetes. Insoluble fibers, found in whole grains, beans, most vegetables, and some fruits, absorb water, making stools softer and bulkier. The names "soluble" and "insoluble" may change in the future to better represent the natural qualities of fiber, but until then, we'll stay with the current naming system.

The Great Energy Providers

When we eat, our bodies only absorb monosaccharide (glucose, fructose, galactose). Fibers are not digested, but soluble fibers can slow the digestive process and add to the feeling of fullness. Soluble fibers also slow the absorption of glucose, which decreases the typical rise in blood sugar levels after eating, which is a big help for patients with diabetes. Foods containing fiber typically have a low Glycemic Index and can minimize the negative effects of foods with a high GI.

For example, according to our dietitian, Anne Dunbar, you can start your day by choosing to eat a healthy, productive breakfast or you can indulge in food that simply drains you of potential energy. That would include foods like sweet rolls or Danish pastry, a large glass of fruit juice, and coffee with white sugar.

What Should We Eat? Carbohydrates 101

I've just described what millions of people slog down on a typical weekday morning. A meal like this—and I use the word "meal" with trepidation—will give you a boost of energy for about 30 to 45 minutes, and then the sugar high will disappear, leaving you feeling tired and sluggish.

On the other hand, you can enjoy the benefits of an energy-reviving breakfast, including an egg white omelet with lots of veggies, whole-grain bread, a piece of fresh fruit, and a cup of non-fat or low-fat milk. A meal like this will last for at least three hours and will provide sustained energy to last you until lunchtime. The blend of protein and complex carbs will maintain your blood sugar at an optimum level, leaving you alert and energized.

Energy-Depleting Breakfast
Plain bagel with butter or cream cheese, sweet roll or Danish pastry, large glass of fruit juice, coffee with white sugar

Energy-Boosting Breakfast
Egg white omelet with veggies,
one slice whole-grain bread,
a piece of fresh fruit,
cup of green tea with half teaspoon of agave syrup

NOTE:
For more breakfast menus, see Chapter 13.

The Chemistry of Good Health

The primary purpose of carbohydrates is to provide our bodies with energy. Our bodies utilize the glucose it derives from the carbohydrates we eat more efficiently than the glucose contained in protein or fat. Carbs and proteins provide about four calories of glucose per gram (whereas fat provides nine calories per gram), but our bodies do not process glucose from proteins quite as smoothly as they do from carbs.

Proteins, however, serve other important functions in our bodies, such as replacing the body's hormones, enzymes, blood cells, and even antibodies. (More on that in the next chapter.) When we eat the appropriate amount of carbohydrates (stay tuned!), we allow our bodies to use the proteins we eat more specifically for their own ideal, special functions. Once our body's energy needs are met, excess glucose can then be used in one of four different ways: creation of glycogen, creation of nonessential amino acids, creation of carbohydrate-containing compounds, and finally, the creation of fat.

What does all this chemistry talk mean?

It's all about glucose and how it affects your body. Remember that sandwich cookie? As you eat it, your body extracts what it needs to meet its immediate energy requirements. The rest settles in your liver or in your muscles as glycogen, or fat. Unlike fat storage, glycogen storage is very limited and is only able to accommodate enough energy for about half a day's worth of moderate activity. Any leftover glucose can be converted into triglycerides and stored in fat cells, where it can remain as fat until the body calls on it for future use.

What Should We Eat? Carbohydrates 101

Here's where things get sticky. If a person has a lot of energy stored as fat, but never needs it because he or she does not lead an active, energy-burning life, then those fat cells are never used up, and they just sit there as those ten pounds of fat you can never seem to lose, no matter how you change your diet. So keep in mind, once you store energy as fat, you have to actively get rid of it.

STOP!

EXERCISE BREAK!

Were you starting to think we forgot? Ha ha. No.
Put down the book and do your top ten!
In fact, let's increase the regimen to 15 minutes.
Start with a little stretching and then bring
out your arsenal of exercises.
When in doubt, go outside and take a jog.
If jogging is an issue, go for a walk.
And keep moving fast enough that
you're not breathing easily.

The Low-Carb Lie

Many of my patients tell me, "Doc, I'm eating healthier, just like you recommended, but I still can't seem to lose weight." Well, you probably already know that in spite of your best intentions, it's difficult to lose weight merely by changing your diet. If you begin today to eat only what your body needs—no more, no less—then you will maintain your current weight. In order to lose weight, you will have to use up what your body has stored as fat.

How do you do that? A low-carb diet, right? It says so on TV so it must be a good thing. Somebody kind of famous is even saying it's good so it must be!

Almost. Like a dream come true, low-carb diets promise salvation, except here's what really happens when you follow that kind of eating plan. If you stay with it long enough, you will deplete your supply of glycogen (stored fat) and the water that's naturally stored along with it, giving you a relatively easy and quick loss of 5 to 10 pounds, depending on your actual body weight. But if you eat anything that replenishes those glycogen stores, you will gain the weight back in a hurry. And by the way, the weight is not actually fat, not literally. It's just water and glycogen! Losing that initial weight doesn't mean you've lost an ounce of fat, despite dropping something like a bowling ball in weight.

Contrary to popular belief, all those diets you hear about are mind games, designed to play with your emotions. The science is this: to lose fat, you have to keep depleting your glycogen storages and force you body to burn the stored fat as a source of energy. Because the body is very good at trying to keep things in balance, weight loss must be a consistent effort to keep your energy output greater than your energy input. Sporadic starts and stops will do nothing lasting for you. Consistency is the only way. Once you reach your target weight, maintaining it becomes easier because adapting and maintaining a steady state of being is what your body does best.

In spite of what we most often read and hear, the fat we eat is much more of a problem in how it applies to our weight than the carbohydrates we eat. The problem we have with too many people in our society is eating too many of the wrong kind of carbohydrates.

Identifying Good Sources of Carbs

Carbohydrates are found in nearly every food group: grains, vegetables, fruits, and even some plants (nuts, beans, and peas). Leading health experts recommend that the majority of the calories in our diet come from "good" carbs, including whole grains, fruits, and vegetables. It is recommended that at least half of our grain intake should be whole grain, and we should vary the grains we eat. The reason to vary is because different whole grains contain different important nutrients, and mixing them allows us to balance the nutrients they provide.

The Dietary Reference Intake (DRI) means that 45 to 65 percent of adult's and children's daily energy intake comes from carbohydrates. The daily amount of carbohydrates a brain needs to function is 130 grams, so that is why the Recommended Dietary Allowance (RDA) for carbohydrates is 130g for adults and children (it is different for infants). For fiber, it is recommended that we consume between 25 to 38 grams per day (based on age and gender).

Let's examine an average serving of some of these foods. For example, one cup of steamed broccoli, a

The Wright Choice

1-ounce slice of bread, 1 medium piece of fruit, or 1 cup of berries is equivalent to 15 grams of carbohydrates. Therefore, in order to accumulate 130 grams of carbohydrates for any given day you need to eat at least two servings of carbohydrates at breakfast, lunch, and dinner (a total of 90 grams) and one serving for a mid-morning snack, one in mid-afternoon, and one last dose in the evening. That will provide an additional 45 grams of carbs. By dividing up your carbohydrates throughout the day, you will insure a steady energy level. To get enough fiber, choose whole-grain breads and cereals and whole fresh fruits. The examples mentioned here provide at least 30 grams of fiber per day.

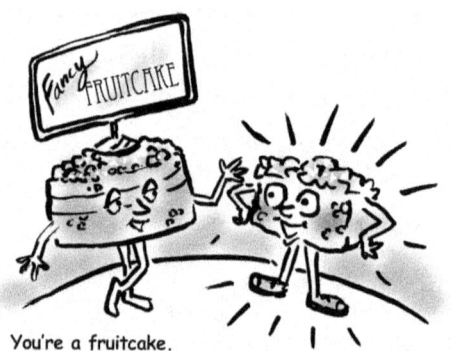

You're a fruitcake.

Yes, but I'm a *very healthy* fruitcake!

Take the Whole-Grain Train!

Bread has gotten a bad reputation in the anti-carb movement. But like with most controversies, there are two sides to the story. It's true that eating any old kind of bread is not wise. As you read on, pay attention to the red flags we're raising about foods with little to no good nutritional value that compromise your body's optimal health. When applying the principals of nutrition to breads, it is easy to see why some should be avoided and some should be sought after.

Grains (the seeds of plants) are the most basic element in bread. A single grain is composed of four basic parts: husk (hull), bran, endosperm, and germ. The husk is the hard protective covering of the seed, which is typically removed because it is inedible. The bran serves as additional layers of protection for the germ and is a source for fiber, B vitamins, niacin, selenium, and pantothenic acid. The endosperm, the starchy part of the grain, made up of protein, carbohydrates, trace minerals, and small amounts of vitamins. The heart of the seed is the germ, which is the source of protein, fat, iron, phosphorus, selenium, potassium, Vitamin E, and thiamin.

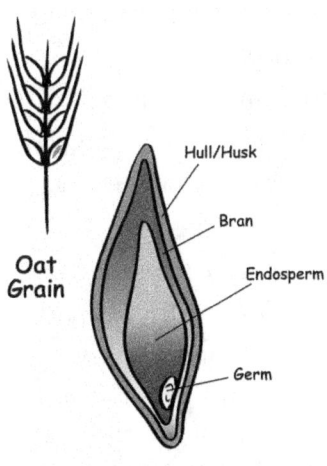

Diagram of a Grain

In the past, grains were consumed whole, with the exception of the husk. Over time, it was found that the bran and germ portions of the grain, which are composed of oils, have a limited shelf life. It was also found that if the bran and the germ layers were removed, the resulting grain was much softer and more appealing. As a result, the refining process began, by removing the bran and germ portions of the grain, and just keeping the endosperm. This refined grain is rich in carbohydrates, but lacks the fiber, vitamins, minerals, and important phytochemicals found in the bran and germ layers of the grain. Eventually, most breadmakers started to bleach their flour with chemicals to make it even more visually appealing, and thus more profitable. It came to be known as white bread.

Wonder Bread is NOT Wonderful!

While whole grains have many benefits, white bread should barely be called food. Your child could eat dirt and enjoy approximately the same nutritional value. It's not that a few slices of well-known white bread will do bad things to you. It's just that it offers your body absolutely no good! Unless you find yourself on a desert island, there are an infinite amount of better options.

Since its inception in 1921, Wonder bread has become an indelible part of our consumer culture. We've seen enough advertising over the years that I'm sure most of us have come to believe that if it's been around so long it *must* be good for us!

What Should We Eat? Carbohydrates 101

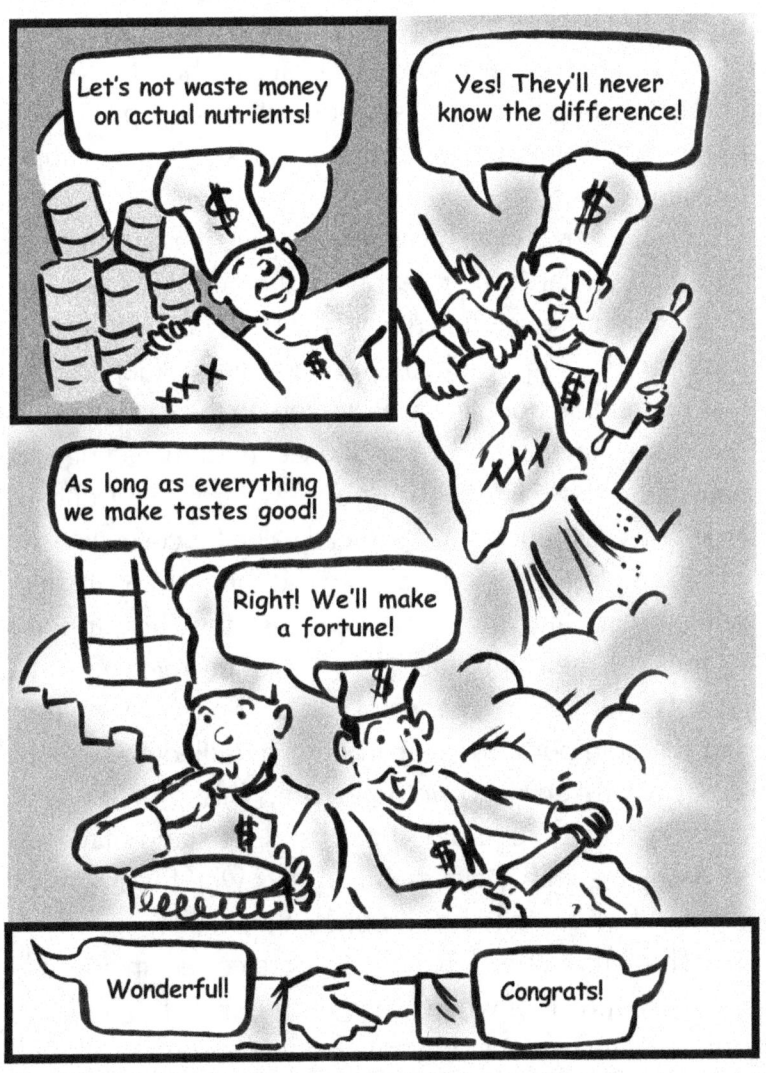

Did you know that you can squeeze a loaf of Wonder bread into a ball the size of your fist? Does that sound like food? Food you want to feed your children? I suppose if you're one of the people who are faithful to certain brands, and you just can't see yourself giving up Wonder bread, may I encourage you to at least buy its whole-wheat product?

Here's why. When bread products are manufactured in a fashion similar to Wonder bread, the nutritious portions of the grain are sacrificed to make the grain last longer, look prettier (supposedly), and taste better (debatable). Not to mention doubling as Play-Doh. In the case of white bread, we Americans became the victim of marketing and have suffered at the hands of our own desire for cheap, long-lasting products (we sacrificed value for convenience).

Examples of refined grain products include white rice, white bread, and white flour. Because they are stripped of most of their nutrients, they are often referred to as "empty calories." Because of the absence of the germ and the bran portions, the carbohydrate-filled endosperm is easily broken down into glucose. This is believed to cause a sharp rise in blood glucose levels and may lead to problems with weight gain. This is why the low-carb diet fad has come to be so popular.

Those proposing low-carb diets are correct in advocating the removal of white bread from our diet, but please note: the important word is WHITE bread, not ALL bread. I propose we modify the statement of a low-carb diet to say that we should avoid "empty" carbs, meaning all white (refined) products. So, in reality, carbs are not our enemy by themselves; "empty" carbs are the culprit.

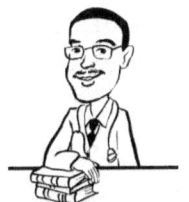

THE WRIGHT ADVICE
The Beauty of Brown Rice

It's not just color that differentiates brown rice from white rice, its processed twin.

Brown rice (long and short grain) is chewier and more nutritious than white rice.

The complete milling and polishing that converts brown rice into white rice destroys 67 percent of the vitamin B3, 80 percent of the vitamin B1, 90 percent of the vitamin B6, half of the manganese, half of the phosphorus, 60 percent of the iron, and all of the dietary fiber and essential fatty acids. It is also known to aid digestion and to be less constipating. The oil in brown rice can help lower cholesterol, prevent heart disease, and reduce the likelihood of getting diabetes.

Health Benefits of Carbohydrates

In its most recent Dietary Guidelines for Americans, the U.S. Department of Health and Human Services reports that individuals who eat generous portions of fruits and vegetables have a decreased risk of developing chronic diseases such as stroke, heart disease, type 2 diabetes, and even certain cancers. The risk of developing coronary heart disease is reduced in individuals who eat foods rich in fiber (fruits, vegetables, and whole-grain products). It also reports that drinking non-fat and low-fat milk can reduce the risk of bone-mass loss over one's lifetime.

On the other side of the coin, too much of a good thing can be bad. Common sense tells us that if we eat too many of the wrong kind of "empty" carbohydrates we can harm our bodies, because too much added sugar can lead to obesity and a multitude of other health problems. But eating too much food—even the right kinds—can lead to unnecessary weight gain, which will present a host of unwanted health issues. Even whole-grain foods, full of fiber and other nutritious elements, can become counterproductive when ingested in great quantities. We need to be aware of how many calories we are consuming and eat just enough to maintain our ideal body weight, or eat less in order to lose the proper amount of weight. We will go into great detail about calories in Chapter 9.

RECOMMENDED CARBS

Whole-wheat flour	Whole-grain breads
Oatmeal and Cheerios	Brown rice
Whole-grain barley	Buckwheat
Quinoa	Millet
Amaranth	Sorghum
Rye	Spelt
Kamut	

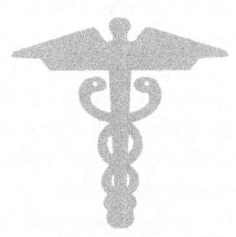

The Wright Reminders

Avoid unnecessary, excessive amounts of sugar.

Eat three or more ounces of whole grains per day.

Eat a variety of fiber-rich fruits and vegetables.

Drink at least three glasses of fat-free milk daily.

Exercise!

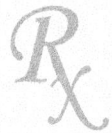

CHAPTER 7
The ABCs of Protein

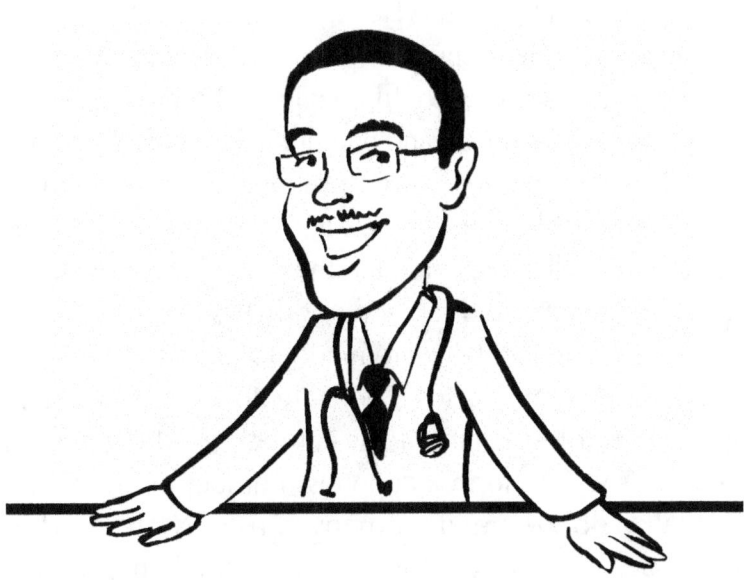

The Essentials

Can you remember back to elementary school when you were first learning to read? The first goal you had to overcome was learning all 26 letters of the alphabet. You most likely memorized them at first, as a result of your parents repeatedly quizzing you. Then you started putting letters together to form words. Words were fun to learn, because each one had a different meaning and allowed you to tell your mom and dad how you felt and what you wanted. Each word served a specific purpose. As you learned more and more of them, you realized that words could express just about anything.

SUPERCALIFRAGILISTICEXPIALIDOCIOUS!

Remember how much fun it was to say that out loud, the longest word you could imagine? The power of language lies in the mental and emotional content that comes with it. When we talk about proteins, think of them as words, essential for our bodies, and how we feel. Proteins are found in all living cells, and their primary role is building, maintaining, and repairing body tissue.

Like words, proteins are made up of smaller components called amino acids. There are 20 amino acids, and like letters, these amino acids can be linked together in countless way to form a countless number of proteins.

Why do we need so many? Proteins are used in cell transport, energy storage, muscle building, muscle contraction, the immune system, blood clotting, hormone creation, and much more.

Of those 20 amino acids, our body can create 11 by itself. That leaves 9 amino acids that our bodies must get through our diet. These are called the essential amino acids, because it is vital that we get these from the foods we eat.

The liver does the all-important role of creating and breaking down proteins. This is a never-ending job, because the body cannot store excess amino acids. All of them must be created on a daily basis, in a process called protein synthesis.

The main role of amino acids is to repair and replace needed proteins. However, under certain conditions, amino acids can be converted into glucose or fat and used for energy. This occurs when there are not enough carbohydrates to support our energy needs, and glycogen stores are used up. This can happen when the body is starved of nutrients and nourishment, or in simple cases of dehydration.

When something like this occurs, it is an expensive and extremely taxing endeavor for the body, because amino acids are now no longer being used to repair and replace our cells. When our bodies begin using amino acids for energy, it is somewhat self-destructive and should be avoided at all costs.

> **STOP!**
>
> **EXERCISE BREAK!**
>
> Before we go any further, it's time for your
> 15-minute (minimum) exercise break.
>
> That will be your first of at least two for the day.
>
> (And it's fine if you want to exercise more.)
>
> Hopefully, you've eaten enough protein to fuel your fun.
>
> If you're hungry when you return, be selective
> about what you choose for a snack.
>
> Avoid fat, salt, and sugar.

Where Does Protein Come From, and What Does It Do?

The first image of protein that pops into most people's minds is beef! Meat, meat, and more meat! For better or worse, we are a carnivorous nation! While it's true that meat is a big source of protein, it's far from the only one. Nearly all foods contain some amount of protein, with the exception of fruits and oils. Sources include grains, nuts, vegetables, dairy products, beans, fish, chicken, soy products, and beef. As you can tell, it's not very hard to get protein in our diet. In fact, studies suggest that the average American diet provides about 50 percent more protein than needed!

Now, not all protein sources are equal in their value. Since the body's reason for eating protein is to acquire amino acids to continue essential bodily functions (whereas our goal may be simply to enjoy a good prime rib steak), the main measure of a protein is the type and amounts of amino acids it provides.

A complete protein contains adequate amounts of all nine of the essential amino acids. Therefore, it's not hard to imagine that a steak may have a different protein count than a pinto bean! With the exception of gelatin, all animal sources of protein are complete. Animal sources include meat, poultry, fish, eggs, and dairy products. The only complete protein from plant sources is soy. Let's look at what each of these protein sources provides and then you can figure out, along with advice from your doctor, what options are best for you and your family. Keep an open mind. Many of you who were brought up to eat a diet dominated by animal products may want to reconsider your normal habits and make some new choices.

Traditional Sources of Protein: Meat, Chicken, and Fish

Whether it's simple hamburgers, steaks, chicken nuggets, or a bagel with lox, most of us have been raised in a culinary tradition that features animal products as our main, if not exclusive, source of protein. That's not altogether bad, by any means. But it's important to know if we are getting enough protein from these sources, or, as I mentioned earlier, we may be actually ingesting too much protein for our systems to effectively manage.

Equally important to consider is how these foods are made and served. Like my friend at the hospital cafeteria, are you eating your hamburger (even made with the best low-fat ground beef) on a roll made from white flour and slathered in a brand of ketchup, which has an unnecessary amount of sugar in it?

Is that supposedly healthy chicken you're serving your family being fried in the skillet with an animal fat, high in saturated fat? Does the breading have any nutritional value? And what about that barbecue sauce you're using? Have you examined its ingredients? (More on reading grocery labels in Chapter 12.)

The same goes for the bagel hosting that protein-filled salmon. Is it made from whole-wheat flour? If you're cooking the salmon on your stovetop, I hope you're not bathing it in butter. For now, let's discover the proteins we can find in milk, cheese, and other dairy products.

Dairy

While dairy products such as milk and cheese can be high in protein, they are not necessarily healthy in other ways. Dairy represents no significant source of fiber, and its fat content needs to be watched. For adults, we recommend non-fat versions of milk, cheese, and yogurts. Children should be drinking 1% fat milk and other dairy products should be low fat. Because flavored milks and ice cream have high fat content and added sugar they should be eaten only on rare occasions.

Vegetarian, Vegan, and Macrobiotic Diets

There is an entire universe of foods available in this world that most people don't yet know about or simply consider too exotic or expensive. For now, let's examine the protein sources we can find in these indisputably healthy alternatives.

Beans and legumes provide plenty of protein and some carbohydrates, as well. Explore how you can add beans (canned are okay and don't require any preparation) to salads, soups, and sauces. You can also mix them into brown rice or whole-grain pasta as a main dish.

There are many soy-based alternatives that look and taste a lot like burgers, sausage, or chicken. Experiment with tofu. The wonderful property of tofu is that it takes on the flavor of whatever you add to it. If you mix tofu into a rich vegetable sauce, it will add texture and soak up the flavor of the sauce. Hummus (pureed chickpeas) is excellent with whole-grain pita bread as a side dish or as a main meal along with a salad.

Medical Myth #6
"If I eat tons of protein, I'll be healthy as an ox."

We already know what can happen if we eat too many carbohydrates. Something equally risky can occur if we overload our body with protein.

Medical research shows that consuming too much protein—more than 30 percent of your total daily caloric intake—could actually harm your body, says protein expert Gail Butterfield, PhD, RD, director of Nutrition Studies at the Palo Alto Veterans' Administration Medical Center and nutrition lecturer at Stanford University. Dr. Butterfield says that adding more protein but not more calories or exercise to your diet won't help you build more muscle mass, but it may put your other bodily systems under stress.

In fact, excessively cutting back on carbohydrates may cause a buildup of toxins in your kidneys, forcing them to work much harder in order to flush them from your body. As a result, you can lose a significant amount of water, which puts you at risk of dehydration, especially if you exercise heavily. While it may appear as if you've lost weight (due to water loss), you may be losing muscle mass and bone calcium. The dehydration also strains your kidneys and puts stress on your heart.

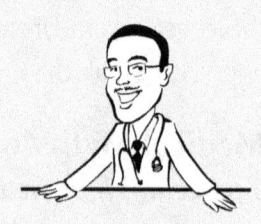

RANDY'S RULES
Consult your doctor or a licensed nutritionist to determine how much protein in your daily diet is best for you.

High Protein Foods from Natural Sources

Eggs (one medium)	6g	Milk (one glass)	6g
Soymilk (one glass)	6g	Tofu (100g serving)	8g
Low-fat yogurt (plain)	8g	Cod filet (one piece)	21g
Cheddar cheese (100g)	25g	Roast beef (100g)	28g
Roast chicken (100g)	25g		

How Much Protein Do I Need?

The amount of protein you require depends on your weight and daily caloric intake. Most Americans consume more than enough protein in their daily diets. A few specific groups of people are at risk for being protein-deficient, including elderly women and people with illnesses or eating disorders. A protein deficiency is defined as eating 50 to 75 percent of the recommended amount of daily protein, Butterfield explains.

Ideally, you should consume 0.36 grams of protein for every pound of body weight, according to recommended daily allowances (RDA) set by the Food and Nutrition Board. For example, if you weigh 170 pounds, you need about 61 grams of protein each day.

Protein should also make up approximately 15 percent of your total daily caloric intake, also according to the RDA. In a diet of 1,800 calories a day, for example, about 270 of those calories should come from protein.

Let's look at the makeup of a variety of protein sources. Ask your doctor what he or she feels is best for you, given your age, size, and general health. It's important that you record how much of these different foods you eat. Knowing what you are eating is the only way you can properly assess your situation. It's the only way your doctor can really help you, too.

Why are there no processed meats (ham, sausage, bacon, bologna, salami, etc.) on the list? The key word is "processed," because we recommend that you stay far away from foods that need to be played with that much before being served or sold. Remember, this book is intended to create healthy families, not sick, chemically treated families getting sicker by the day. OUCH!

As you gather information on the merits of eating meat versus the benefits of a vegetarian diet, it's understandable that you may be confused. Advertising doesn't help either. We see people—with uncommonly "perfect" physiques—promoting the use of specific supplements and formulas, while on the other hand you might be wondering if the yoga center opening up in your neighborhood next to the health food store might be the healthy way to go. Who's right and what path should we take? Let's look at the pros and cons of each group.

The Meat Eaters

In this camp, meat is king, and it serves as the main source of protein. Most Americans fall into this group, eating about 50 percent more protein than they need. The typical meal is centered around a particular portion of meat, with a little bit of green stuff (vegetable garnish) sprinkled around it to make us feel good. The problem with this group is portion control and fat intake. The Recommended Dietary Allowance (RDA) for protein is 10 percent of the total calories. For most of us, that steak that takes up 70 percent of the plate is a little too much protein.

The good thing about diets featuring animal products is that they are mainly complete sources of protein (besides gelatin). However, diets heavily dependent on animal products may be high in fat content, specifically saturated and trans fats, which increase the risk of heart disease, stroke, and certain cancers. For this reason, the American Heart Association suggests a balanced diet low in fat, emphasizing whole grain, fruits, and vegetables.

The Plant Eaters

In this group, plants are king, and avoiding meat is the rule. The general name for this group is vegetarian, and people choose this path because of religion, politics, or health.

Studies now show that plant-based diets may in fact be healthier than those based primarily on animal products. Variations on the vegetarian diet include those who eat only plant products (vegans), those whose diet includes plants plus dairy products (lacto vegetarians), and those who eat plants, milk products, and eggs (lacto-ovo vegetarians).

But being a vegetarian takes work, especially when it comes to getting enough of the proper sources of protein, providing the essential amino acids to avoid malnutrition. It is also important to avoid sources of protein that are high in fat and cholesterol (whole milk, eggs, and cheeses, for example).

The Fish Eaters

Seafood is a great source of protein and omega-3s. The fattier the fish, the more beneficial fatty acids it has to protect your heart. The American Heart Association (AHA) lists mackerel, lake trout, salmon, sardines, herring, and albacore tuna as the highest in omega-3s. The AHA says that shrimp and crawfish are higher in cholesterol than most fish, but lower in saturated fat and total fat than most meats and poultry. Just make sure that your seafood choices are not fried, dipped in butter, or prepared with other fat. For example, a bowl of boiled shrimp with red sauce makes a healthy appetizer or a meal. In Chapter 13, we provide many recipes for you to incorporate into your diet.

Invasion of the Shake People

Fitness centers and nutrition companies claim that building muscle requires more protein. For those who believe this, extra protein may come in the form of shakes, supplements, and extra servings of animal products. The reality is that more is not necessarily better, needed, and may even be harmful, especially when taken in the wrong amounts.

It takes an extra two ounces of meat (14 grams of protein) per day to gain one pound of muscle in one week. This is not much, and considering that the average American diet includes 50 percent more protein than we need, eating a high-protein diet is not necessary, because most people already get plenty of protein.

Taking specific amino acids and protein drinks is not necessarily a good idea. Since the body must have all 20 amino acids present in order to build proteins, being overstocked in a few areas and under stocked in others serves only to prevent protein production. Also, some experts believe that high-protein diets consumed over a long period of time may lead to kidney damage. So, for muscle building, the best advice is old-fashioned exercise and adequate amounts of calories and protein.

Can I Eat Too Much Protein?

You certainly can. According to the American Heart Association, most Americans already ingest more protein than they require. That means, depending on how much protein they're eating, they may be risking their health. Too much protein in your diet that comes from red meat sources also increases the amount of saturated fat and cholesterol you eat. This puts you at an elevated risk for coronary heart disease, diabetes, stroke, and several types of cancer. Those people who can't process excess proteins effectively in their bodies can also be at higher risk for kidney and liver disorders, and in some cases, osteoporosis.

How to Be Protein Friendly for Your Body

Let's assume you're reading this book because you want to put yourself and your family on a better path to good health. But at the same time, it's hard to give up those old habits, right? So, you may be asking, what about a mixed diet of red meat and vegetarian food? Of course! The rules you make should be rules you can keep. Otherwise, they simply become a steady succession of goals you can't reach, and eventually you'll just stop trying. Let's be realistic. You want to keep eating hamburgers and steak. Can't go too long without that pork chop. Understood. But there's a way you can treat yourself better and still enjoy those foods.

It begins with selective shopping. Purchase the highest quality meat you can afford. Lean cuts, organic beef, kosher meat, and grass-fed products top the list of what's best for you. In normal commercial markets, look for lean fat versions in the meat department. For example, ground beef can often be purchased at different percentages of fat. You can usually find it at 90 percent lean or even higher. Tell the attendant your concerns and ask for his or her recommendation.

How you prepare your food is also crucial. Let's agree from the start that you're going to keep your frying pan off the stovetop as much as possible. Sure, it's convenient to throw some meat in a frying pan and serve it up, but the amount of fat you use to fry it, and what happens to the food while it goes through the frying process is not what you really want for your family. The healthier alternative is broiling or baking.

Meat As a Side Dish

While we're at it, let's go a step further and challenge you with the concept of eating meat as a side dish in your main menu. For example, let's look at a nice dinner of spaghetti (whole-wheat or spinach mixed in with the "normal" type), accompanied by a tomato sauce with fresh vegetables, and a mixed salad with a modest amount of dressing (more on that in Chapter 13).

That leaves us with our main dish, which might often be meat. How about switching that up, and on the nights you aren't already serving a main dish of chicken or fish, try adding vegetables, beans, and tofu and using a small serving of meat as an accent? Instead of a ten-ounce steak to dominate the plate, how about a broccoli soufflé and 4 ounces of broiled steak? You get the best of both worlds this way. Your overall calorie count is good, you're conserving fat and using carbohydrates properly, and still indulging your taste for a good old-fashioned steak. Everybody wins.

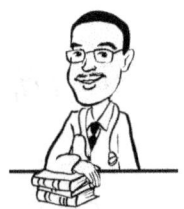

THE WRIGHT ADVICE

Please take a moment to visit the website of
the American Heart Association
for more information about eating meat as a side dish.

www.heart.org

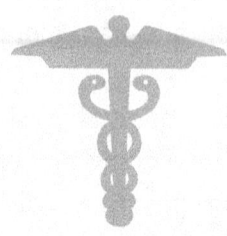

The Wright Reminders

Evaluate the amount of protein in your diet.

Identify its sources.

Make necessary adjustments.

Try new sources of protein.

Serve meat as a side dish.

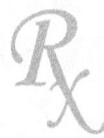

CHAPTER 8

It's a
Fat Fat Fat Fat World

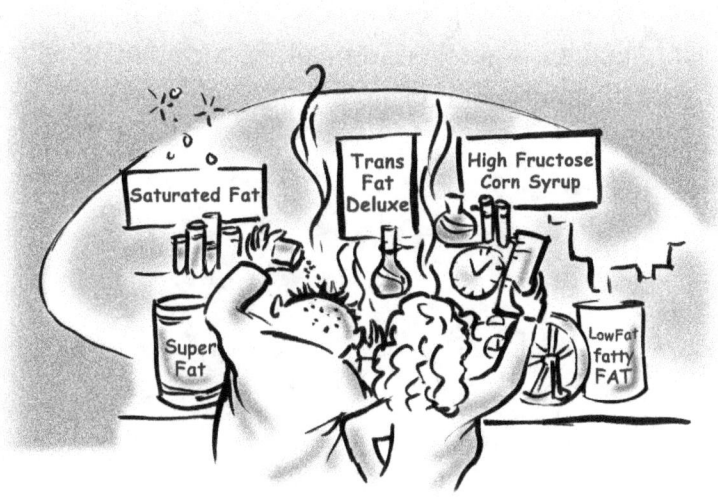

The Skinny on Fats

In the opening scene of *It's a Mad Mad Mad Mad World*, Jimmy Durante, playing a crook who has robbed a tuna factory, reveals where he hid an enormous stash of cash. Five different bystanders take off simultaneously in pursuit of the money. So begins a hilarious portrayal of basic human greed. The message is, if something looks too good to be true, it probably is.

The same can be said for fat, as in the food we eat.

The problem with fat is that for most people, it tastes sooooooo good, and we really want to eat it. It has been used to cook almost anything: fried shrimp, fried fish, deep-fried oysters, French fries, ice cream, pizza, fried okra, tempura, and the list goes on. Fats are so engrained in our culture that it is sometimes difficult for most people to list 10 foods that do not contain a significant amount of fat.

> **STOP!**
>
> **EXERCISE BREAK!**
>
> While you're trying to come up with that list,
> it's time for your 20-minute exercise break.
>
> You read that correctly—20 minutes.
>
> That'll burn off some of the fat you've eaten so far today.
>
> And remind you not to eat too much more!
>
> In fact, after you burn off some calories over
> the next 20 minutes, pay attention to what
> kind of snack you have afterward.

Addicted to Fat?

As Americans, it's possible that we are addicted to fat. We cook foods with fat, we like how it tastes, we buy foods that are fatty; grocery stores, restaurants, and fast-food chains then started to provide us with more fatty foods. Over time, since we tend to prefer fatty foods more than non-fatty foods, the majority of the food on the market became fatty. So now, when we want to start eating healthy, it's hard, because healthy alternatives are harder to find. The market is driven by consumers who want fatty foods so that's what stores sell. So now fatty foods are cheaper and more accessible, and eating healthy is harder and more expensive for most.

"Eat less fat!"

Unless you have been living under a rock for the past 50 years, you have heard this statement endlessly from numerous experts. But do you really do it, and do you really know why? Like most things in life, there are no absolutes, and details are important. With fat, it is completely unfair to say, "All fat is bad." In fact, fat is an essential part of life. There are many different types of "fat," and our bodies need these various forms in order to function properly. For example, cholesterol is essential to the production of certain hormones, bile acids, cell membranes, and even vitamin D. Omega-3 fatty acids are important regulators of blood pressure, blood clotting, and even metabolism of triglycerides!

The Good, the Bad, and the Saturated

A recurring theme that you may see is that there are no absolutes: there is no one perfect diet, there is no one drug to cure all ills, and all fats are not necessarily bad. We cannot talk about the bad things of fat without talking about the good things fatty acids provide.

The good fats are the unsaturated fats. These are fatty acids that do not have all the hydrogen atoms attached to them that they could potentially hold. Because of this, double bonds exist between the carbon atoms that are present. If a fatty acid has one double bond, it is called a monounsaturated fatty acid. If two or more double bonds exist, it is called a polyunsaturated fatty acid. The number of double bonds in a fatty acid determines, in part, its structure. The more double bonds, the more kinked (curved) the molecule is.

This kinking, as we learned earlier, prevents the fatty acid molecule from stacking tightly and this results in the fat becoming a liquid at room temperature. Examples include oils and soft margarines. Unsaturated fatty acids also go bad sooner than saturated fats when exposed to light and oxygen. Examples of monounsaturated fatty acids include canola, olive, and peanut oil. Examples of polyunsaturated fatty acids include omega-6 polyunsaturated fatty acids and omega-3 polyunsaturated oils. Omega-6 polyunsaturated fatty acids can be found in plant oils such as soybean, sunflower, corn, and cottonseed. Sources of omega-3 polyunsaturated oils include fish oils such as salmon, trout, herring, mackerel, and swordfish. Some plant oils that contain omega-3s include flaxseed, hazelnuts, canola, and even walnuts. Unsaturated fats are considered positive fats because they provide us with some health benefits. If eaten in place of saturated fats, monounsaturated fats may lower LDL cholesterol levels. Omega-3s have been found to protect the heart by lowering LDL and by other means. Exactly how these fatty acids decrease the risk of heart disease is still being studied, but research suggests they may decrease triglyceride levels, lower blood pressure slightly, slow the growth rate of plaque buildup in arteries, and possibly even lower the risk of deadly heart rhythms that can lead to heart attacks.

The "Bad Boys" of Food

Why does it always seem like our favorite actors are the Hollywood "Bad Boys" and "Bad Girls." Those individuals who are so tempting and give us guilty pleasure in watching them work. Why was it that we always seemed to fall for the wrong person early on in the dating scene? It seems like I can still remember my mother telling me that "beauty is more than skin deep" and "all that glitters is not gold."

Boy, was she right.

How many times did I see my friends fall head over heels for a hot girl, only to learn that she was more trouble than she was worth? How many times have I had female friends in college confide in me that they found a guy who drove a great car, bought them wonderful things, and was so much fun to be with only to turn out to be a jerk? Luckily, most of these friends eventually made the right choice and are now happily married. I raise this point because I see many similarities in early dating and eating. When we are relatively new to the dating scene, we are fascinated with exciting, fun, and over-the-top individuals, often the ones mom wouldn't approve of. However, after lots of trial and error, we learn (hopefully) that the Bad Boy or Bad Girl type is mostly smoke and mirrors and not at all worth our time.

We actually mature with age and realize that there is more to a relationship than sly conversation and late-night rendezvous. We learn that true happiness is rooted in finding a companion who shares similar interests, life's goals, and spiritual beliefs. The exciting things should be there, but they may take a back burner to less flashy qualities that actually add value to our lives.

The same is true with food. In today's society we are addicted to convenience, speed, and pleasure. Many of the food choices we make are based on easy access and appeal. Nutritional value for many people is an afterthought at best. This food-choice behavior is like falling for the Bad Boy or Bad Girl mother warned us about. Many of us eat to please taste first and if it is nutritious, then that's an added bonus. The foods that tend to qualify in this category are typically high in fat. So let's learn about the foods that mother should have warned us about, and why they are bad.

Bad Fats: Trans and Hydrogenated

On April 18, 1775, Paul Revere did his now famous midnight ride from Boston to Lexington, Massachusetts, warning the colonists that the British were coming. I predict a trans fat revolution in the upcoming years, so let this book serve as a warning. "The trans fats are coming! The trans fats are coming!"

We can no longer keep our heads in the dark and believe that it does not matter what we eat. Trans fats are the essence of the Bad Boy that looks good but will really get you into trouble.

To understand trans fat, we have to turn to the food manufacturing industry. Americans like products that taste good, can be eaten or prepared quickly, and can last a long time without going bad. Trans fats became the answer to that request, but at a price.

Around the turn of the twentieth century, the process of hydrogenation was discovered, a process in which curved polyunsaturated fatty acids are made straight by adding hydrogen molecules. Polyunsaturated fats are liquid at room temperature because their curved or "kinked" structure prevents them from stacking together tightly to form a solid substance. Hydrogenation fixed this problem and allowed food manufacturers to create solid, longer lasting substances that actually had an appealing taste and texture.

The commercial food industry loved this process. In 1911, Procter & Gamble introduced Crisco vegetable shortening, the first man-made product containing trans fats. Many similar products followed, such as stick margarine and shortening.

The health problems trans fats presented did not become evident (at least to the public) until many years later. In 1957, the American Heart Association first proposed a reduction in consumption of foods containing saturated fats. As time passed, the truth about hydrogenation became clear, and in 2006 it became law for food labels to list their respective amounts of trans fats. The AHA became the first organization to specify a daily limit of trans fats in a person's diet, recommending that less than 1 percent of calories come from trans fats.

It's a Fat Fat Fat Fat World

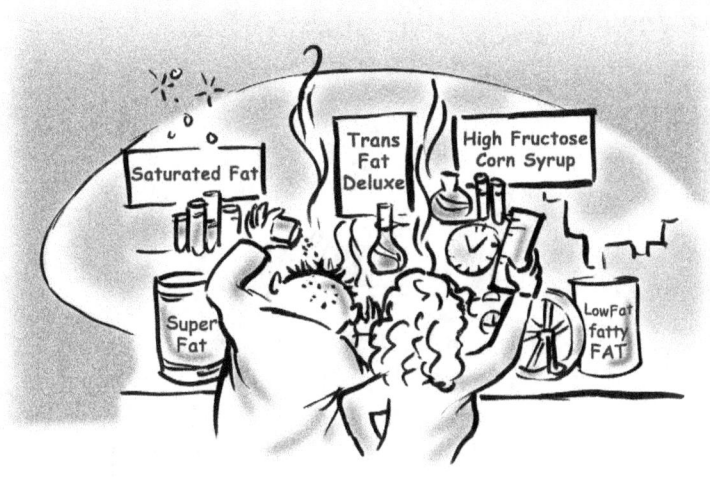

Today, trans fats, despite their known health risks, continue to appear in many foods, such as stick margarines, shortenings, many deep-fried products, French fries, pie crusts, doughnuts, pastries, pizza dough, biscuits, cookies, and crackers.

Wow, that seems like all the fun foods we like to eat! Therefore, I repeat the point that our fascination (or addiction as some authorities may argue) with fatty foods is the equivalent of falling in love with the one your mother warned you about. It seems fun at the time, but you will probably get hurt and become unhappy later! What's so sexy about a Big Mac or a 99-cent taco, anyway?

The American Heart Association recommends eliminating trans fats from our diet and significantly reducing saturated fats. They suggest that we eat fatty fish (such as salmon, albacore tuna, mackerel, lake trout, sardines, and even herring) at least twice a week.

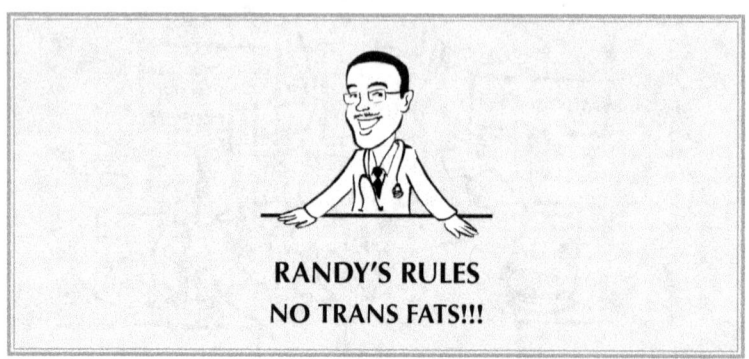

**RANDY'S RULES
NO TRANS FATS!!!**

Saturated Fat

At its most basic level, a fatty acid is a chain of carbon atoms with hydrogen atoms attached to it. A saturated fatty acid (saturated fat for short) is a fatty acid where all of the carbon atoms are bonded to the maximum number of hydrogen atoms it can hold. Literally it is "saturated" with hydrogen atoms. Because of this, they are typical straight molecules, which make them able to stack on top of one another very easily. This stackable ability is what makes saturated fats solid at room temperature. They are also very stable and do not turn bad as quickly as the unsaturated fats. For these reasons, they are favorites in the kitchen. Saturated fats can be found in animal meats, dairy products, and certain tropical oils, such as coconut and palm kernel.

Foods that contain a significant amount of saturated fats include beef, lamb, chicken with the skin, pork, cheese, whole milk, and even 2% milk. What makes saturated fats bad for us is that they raise our levels of LDL cholesterol, which, as we learned earlier, increase our risk for heart attack and stroke.

The American Heart Association recommends that we keep our daily consumption of saturated fats to less than 7 percent of our daily intake. So the next time you reach for that double meat burger with cheese, just stop and think for a minute about all of the saturated fats you are about to unleash into your body and what it will do to your arteries.

Medical Myth #7
All Milk Is Good for You

Whole milk derives about half its calories from fat. Reduced-fat milk (2%) derives 35 percent of its calories from fat. Drinking 2% milk is a good way to wean oneself from whole milk, but is too high in fat as a permanent choice, unless your diet is otherwise very low in fat. Low-fat milk (1%) gets 23 percent of its calories from fat.

Many people find low-fat milk more appealing and a good compromise. Skimmed milk/non-fat milk derives just 5 percent of its calories from fat. Skimmed milk has about half the calories of whole milk. It is the best choice for adults, and is the only type of milk that should be consumed by people on strict low-fat diets.

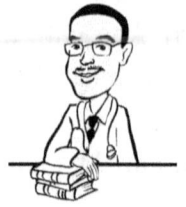

THE WRIGHT ADVICE
Baby Milk Alert

In 2008, The American Academy of Pediatrics changed its recommendation that weaned babies be fed whole milk until they're two years old. It now recommends reduced-fat (2%) milk for those between 12 months and two years of age. After their second birthday, all kids should be switched to low-fat (1%) milk.

Cholesterol: The Good, the Bad, and the Confusing

When we look at health statistics in America, the number-one killer has been, and still is, heart disease. One of the leading risk factors for heart disease is high cholesterol. So any conversation about our health is incomplete if cholesterol is not thoroughly discussed.

Cholesterol is a waxy, fat-like substance that is found naturally in our bodies. Our liver—or other cells—produces approximately 75 percent of it. The remaining 25 percent comes from the foods we eat. Because cholesterol is essential for so many bodily functions, such as maintaining cell membranes, production of bile, production of steroid hormones (cortisol and aldosterone), and even metabolism of the fat-soluble vitamins, it's quite necessary for our existence. However, like most things in life, too much of a good thing can be bad.

High cholesterol levels can be dangerous. Many diets fail to discuss this. They tend to focus only on one number: your weight! While some programs may help you lose weight, they don't necessarily help you live longer by eating healthier. Some replace high-calorie foods with ones lower in calories, but higher in fat, which, as you just learned, literally puts your life at risk for heart attacks or strokes. A good diet plan pays attention to both your caloric intake and your fat intake.

Healthy Cholesterol Range
Total Cholesterol: less than 200 mg/dL
HDL Cholesterol: 60 mg/dL and above
LDL Cholesterol: less than 100 mg/dL optimal
LDL Cholesterol: 100–129 mg/dL near optimal

Borderline Cholesterol Range
Total Cholesterol: 200–239 mg/dL
HDL Cholesterol: 40–50 mg/dL for men
and 50–60 mg/dL for women
LDL Cholesterol: 130–159 mg/dL

High-Risk Cholesterol Range
Total Cholesterol: 240 mg/dL and higher
HDL Cholesterol: below 40 mg/dL in
men and 50 mg/dL in women
LDL Cholesterol: 160–189 mg/dL high
LDL Cholesterol: 190 mg/dL or above very high

Atherosclerosis: Hardening of Whose Arteries?

Cholesterol is like gas. Some of it is necessary for our economy to flourish. But just like at the pumps, there is more than one type of cholesterol. LDL is like the inexperienced driver who often crashes or never makes it to his or her destination. HDL is like the very experienced driver who never crashes and always gets the vehicle from one place to another, and rather quickly, I might add. On this superhighway, the goal is to transport gas, an important commodity for society, from point A to point B. The road, however, is dangerous, and it takes experienced drivers to transport the gas safely.

When times are good, and business is prosperous, HDLs are the predominant choice, ensuring that the roads are typically free of accidents, with traffic running smoothly, and the need for road repair at a minimum. When this is the case, gas flows, and we have a healthy economy. But sometimes the LDL transport system becomes the predominant means used for transporting gas. When this happens, accidents occur due to how LDLs maneuver the road, and there's a potential for a lot of harm. If this continues for long, there may be permanent damage, and some roads will eventually become permanently blocked.

The world inside our arteries is very similar. Cholesterol is the precious cargo essential for proper health. It is insoluble in blood, so it has to be carried by another entity (LDL or HDL). Because it is needed in various parts of the body, it must be transported from the liver to those parts. When used in high amounts, the LDL transport system can lead to damaged blood vessels, and often to clots inside the vessel, which can eventually become blocked, causing a heart attack or a stroke.

This narrowing of a blood vessel is called atherosclerosis. Individuals with high LDL readings are at an increased risk. Conversely, people with high HDL readings and low

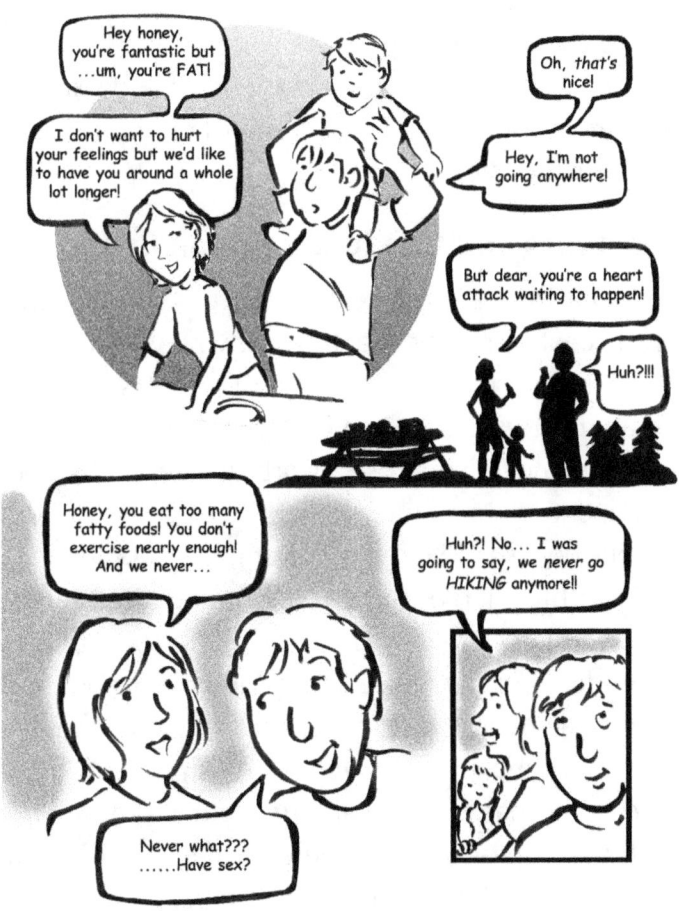

LDL have a reduced risk. The higher your overall cholesterol level, the more likely your LDL level will be too high. While cholesterol by itself is not bad, it's the method of transport (LDL or HDL) that gives it the potential for harm. Many experts believe that HDL is good because it carries cholesterol out of the bloodstream to the liver for excretion. All of them agree that too much LDL is a recipe for disaster.

Are you at risk? Is someone you love walking a tightrope? In either case, you can do yourself and your loved one a great favor by shining a spotlight on the problem—before it's too late.

Sometimes You *Can* Judge a Book By Its Cover

No one can argue with the importance of self-esteem and being accepted in society at large for who you are. But the fact is—and all of medical science will back this up—people who are overweight are more susceptible to a number of afflictions, including stroke, heart disease, and diabetes, not to mention premature death.

Let's be clear. We're not referring to people who are just plain big—large framed, big boned, and generally husky. Genetics are genetics. And we're sorry that most airlines don't make their seats any larger to accommodate nature. In all honesty, we're really talking about those who are proportionately overweight to a significant degree, to the point that it's clinically unhealthy and downright dangerous. Unfortunately, there are far too many men, women, and children in this category.

While we agree with the National Association to Advance Fat Acceptance that people of all sizes and shapes should not be discriminated against, we'd also love to see this group become obsolete, just like we'd love the day to come when we won't need stroke clinics and when I no longer get any 2 a.m. phone calls about an acute stroke in the ER.

The NAAFA claims that more than 65 million people in America are labeled "obese." I'll bet that most of those men, women, and children are not as healthy as they could be. That's what I'd like to be a part of changing. Of course, it's everyone's civil right to be accepted for who he is, but it's also our obligation as good citizens and medical practitioners to inspire people to become more healthy and more involved in their own well-being.

Helping Your Kids Choose Wisely

Personal health and appearance can be a touchy subject between spouses. But let's hope two adults can act like it by examining their lifestyle for their own good. Even so, being honest can be painful. But it's necessary if we want to improve our health.

Imagine then what it's like to confront your own child about his or her bad health habits. First, you must look at your own behavior. Are you a good role model? If so, how can you inspire your child? If not, if you need as much of a makeover as he or she does, then perhaps you can do it together, as a team.

Dr. Mark Banschick, noted child and adolescent psychiatrist and co-author of *The Intelligent Divorce,* recommends that parents, "work on themselves, and by proxy, encourage their children to do the same. We all have weaknesses, and parenting does not require perfection. But if you have a weight problem or smoke, your child will almost certainly follow suit. Show them that you care about taking care of your body and they will be inspired. Have a positive attitude and show them that self-responsibility is something that you value."

According to Me

"Our 14-year-old son, Nate, is new at his school and he's been hanging out with a bunch of boys after soccer practice, hoping to become friends with them. One day, on the way to McDonald's, Nate gets nervous because he's been a vegetarian his entire life.

As a child, his eating habits posed no problems.

Now, as a teenager, everything is an issue. He agrees with the reasons for being a vegetarian, but he's a normal kid and wants to be like everyone else. As he approached the counter to order, he didn't know what to do. Everyone was ordering a Big Mac and fries, and he didn't want to stick out like a sore thumb and possibly be ostracized.

Finally, Nate ordered a milkshake, mumbling something about not being hungry, which he definitely was. Luckily, he said, no one questioned him about it."

Jen, age 51, Jacksonville, Florida

Conversely, if you, the grown-up, insist on continuing the bad habits you've built up over your lifetime, is it any surprise when you see your kids follow suit? If you don't care, why should they? Do you really want to live with that? You'll all pay for it down the road, in increased costs for medical care, lost wages, a compromised lifestyle, and a shortened life expectancy.

When it comes to our children's health, the parent-child dynamic is crucial, but it's only one piece of the puzzle. Peer pressure, especially for teenagers, can be tremendous, and more often than not, our kids are left to their own devices.

DocSpeak

Peer pressure is notorious for causing kids to make poor judgments. Nate wants to be accepted like every kid does, and he should feel secure in his choice of being a vegetarian. In fact, he may end up educating his new friends and doing them a big favor by reconsidering their appetite for fast foods. He doesn't have to preach about not eating meat; he can merely mention his desire to be healthy and in the best shape possible for sports. In fact, a vegetarian diet may not be the optimal choice for everyone. Perhaps Nate can do a bit of online research and find out what famous soccer players are vegetarians. Name-dropping like that can surely bolster his assertion that a healthy diet is worth adhering to. That list gets even bigger, too, when you add in Hollywood actors, musicians, and Olympic athletes.

If You Can't Eliminate—Moderate!

"Eat not to dullness; drink not to elevation," said Benjamin Franklin. Not bad advice. With that in mind, we're certainly not asking anyone to go to any extremes, like giving up 100 percent of your guilty pleasures.

That is, except for smoking. Do whatever is necessary to quit that immediately. If you have children, which you probably do if you're reading this book, get a grip on being a parent and stop smoking right now! How can you even consider smoking when it means you could get sick or die prematurely, leaving your children without a healthy mother or father, or without a parent at all? If you're scoffing at this, even for a second, then you're simply in denial. Smoking hurts you. It even kills. Every adult living in the modern, civilized world knows that. So stop smoking now.

End of lecture.

Back in reality, where we hope you are residing most of the time, it's clear that we all struggle to find an acceptable balance between indulgence and discipline. Smoking (this is merely an afterthought to the lecture), simply because it's bad for you will only indulge a death wish. Discipline, on the other hand, can win you a longer, healthier life. I'm pretty sure that this is desirable for 99.9 percent of the human population.

But back to acknowledging our human frailty. I like ice cream, the real stuff, full of cream and calories and fat, just like the next person, but I have cut down—way down—on the amount of full-fat, high-calorie, some would say toxic, ice cream I ingest. When I have the urge, I opt for low-fat ice cream, or better still, frozen yogurt, or even better, a soy product. They taste just about as good as the guilty pleasure. But don't think I've eliminated old-fashioned ice cream altogether. I limit it to birthdays: my own, my wife's, and my two kids'. That's four times a year I get to indulge. It's quite enough, as it turns out.

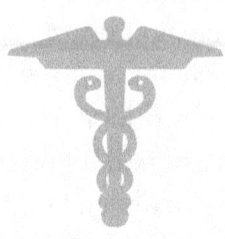

The Wright Reminders

Eat less fat!

No trans fats!

Reduce your daily consumption of saturated fats.

Check your cholesterol every year.

Help your kids make healthy food choices.

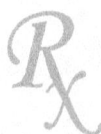

CHAPTER 9

It's All About Calories, Knucklehead

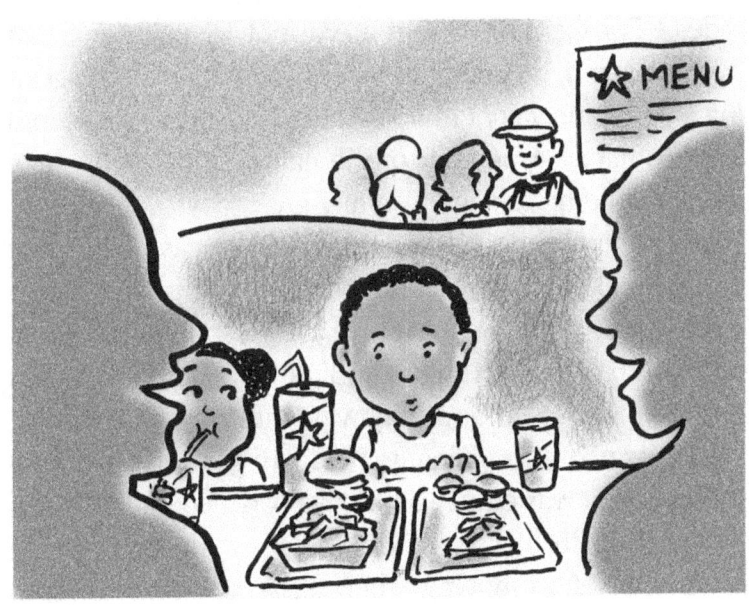

What's a Calorie?

We typically associate the word calorie with measuring how many of them there are in any given food. In fact, a calorie is a unit of energy, specifically, how much energy, or heat, is required to raise the temperature of one gram of water exactly one degree Celsius, or 1.8 degrees Fahrenheit. In the world of chemistry and physical science, one calorie is equivalent to 4.184 joules, the given unit of energy used by scientists.

The *Cambridge International Dictionary of English* defines a food calorie as "a unit of energy, used as a measurement for the amount of energy which food provides." For example, there are about 50 calories in an average apple, meaning if you eat one you will be ingesting energy equivalent to 50 calories, which translates into approximately 4 percent of the caloric total an average adult should be taking in on any given day.

To simplify this further, consider the gas tank in my car. When I fill it with a certain amount of gasoline, it provides energy for my car to drive a corresponding amount of miles, based upon speed and traffic conditions. When I'm driving on a smooth highway with no traffic my car uses energy quite efficiently. But if I'm stuck in city traffic for an hour, I waste quite a bit of valuable energy. To carry the analogy further, if I allow my gas tank to hit empty my car will stop moving. Then again, if I fill it with too much gasoline, it will overflow onto the side of my car

It's All About Calories, Knucklehead

and probably my hand, as well, rendering both of them smelly and flammable. Not to mention that I've wasted money on unused gasoline.

The point is, calories in your body are like gasoline in your car. We want them both to function at their best, using a healthy amount of energy in an efficient manner.

Here's where your body and your car differ. When you don't use up the gas in your tank, it pretty much sits there, waiting for you to use it the next time you drive. Your body works differently. When you eat, your body uses the energy in the particular foods you ingest for things like moving around, thinking, and growing—all the things you do that require energy. But here's the catch: your body stores the energy it doesn't need today and keeps it for the future. It keeps it in your body in the form of fat cells.

If you stay active, the body uses up the energy you feed it with the food you eat. If you sit around too long, reading this book for example, your body will store that energy and those fat cells translate into weight gain. Ouch! We don't want that. Therefore, here are some simple solutions to making your calorie intake work for you and not against you.

Why Math Matters

In 2008, the city of New York became the first city in the United States to pass legislation requiring chain restaurants to post calorie counts on food they are selling. According to the National Restaurant Association, San Francisco, California and King County, Washington, are the only other municipalities in the country that currently have similar laws.

Many towns and cities have defeated efforts to require this information to be made available for its citizens. Why? Because lobbyists representing major food chains have done a highly effective job for their clients who frankly don't want diners to know the details of what they are eating. If they did, it would affect the restaurants' profits, and that would be a disaster! Meanwhile, these food chains are doing everything they can to fatten up Americans at the expense of their own health.

It doesn't have to be that way for you or your family. You can take responsibility for what you eat and how many calories you ingest. The formulas exist. The information is readily available and you need only a little bit of time to learn about it.

The amount of calories an individual needs on a daily basis is determined by using a variety of mathematical formulas. Age, height, and weight all play a role. That is, your present weight and the weight you'd like to be at.

The Unites States Department of Agriculture offers a wealth of information revolving around the basics of the food pyramid. By entering your age, sex, weight, height, and amount of daily physical activity (don't lie!) you will

It's All About Calories, Knucklehead

be provided with a blueprint for healthy eating, including specific amounts of grains, vegetables, fruits, milk, and beans you should be eating each day. It even includes recommended portions of dark green vegetables, orange vegetables, dry beans and peas, starchy vegetables, and others.

Visit www.mypyramid.gov and click on "My Pyramid Plan."

STOP!

EXERCISE BREAK!

Who wants to burn calories?

We know that you do because now that you know about storing fat when you're sitting around, you're ready to make the right choice!

Okay. It's time for your 20-minute (minimum) exercise break.

That'll burn off some calories.

See if you can push yourself this time to go a little further and/or a little harder.

If it takes you 5 minutes to run around the block, see if you can do it in 4:45.

Raise the bar a little bit higher each time.

You're capable of more than you think.

How Many Calories Will I Burn Reading This Chapter?

Now that you've done your exercise—if you haven't then do it now—you can get back to reading this book and burning two calories per minute doing so. If you get hungry reading about food, go in your kitchen and start cooking, burning off calories at three per minute while preparing your family's dinner. If the ironing is piling up, why not take 20 minutes to finish it off, burning 80 calories in the process. Or, when your son gets home from school, why not get a basketball and shoot around with him, burning seven calories a minute, that is, unless you stand at the foul line the entire time. If you play some heated one-on-one, you'll be burning as many as 12 calories per minute. You'd be surprised how many daily activities provide opportunities for burning calories in productive and fun ways. It still amazes me how many of my patients simply forget this, while they remain mysteriously glued to their cars and remote controls. By the way, driving burns calories at three per minute, while you can simmer off two calories per minute watching TV.

The American Heart Association chart on the next page breaks down how many calories are spent per hour during a variety of movement and sports-based activities. Of course, we recommend that you pursue these types of activities because they are more physical and get your metabolism moving in the right direction.

Estimated Calorie Requirements (in kilocalories) for Each Gender and Age Group at Three Levels of Physical Activity

Gender	Age (years)	Sedentary	Activity Level Moderately Active	Active
Child	2–3	1,000	1,000–1,400	1,000–1,400
Female	4–8	1,200	1,400–1,600	1,400–1,800
Female	9–13	1,600	1,600–2,000	1,800–2,000
Female	14–18	1,800	2,000	2,400
Female	19–30	2,000	2,000–2,200	2,400
Female	31–50	1,800	2,000	2,200
Female	51+	1,600	1,800	2,000–2,200
Male	4–8	1,400	1,400–1,600	1,600–2,000
Male	9–13	1,800	1,800–2,200	2,000–2,600
Male	14–18	2,200	2,400–2,800	2,800–3,200
Male	19–30	2,400	2,600–2,800	3,000
Male	31–50	2,200	2,400–2,600	2,800–3,000
Male	51+	2,000	2,200–2,400	2,400–2,800

Source: HHS/USDA Dietary Guidelines for Americans

Calorie Burn Chart

Activity	Calories burned per hour		
	100 lb.	150 lb.	200 lb.
Walking, 2 mph	160	240	312
Walking, 4.5 mph	295	440	572
Running 5.5 mph	440	660	962
Running, 10 mph	850	1,280	1,664
Swimming, 25 yds/min	185	275	358
Swimming, 50 yds/min	325	500	650
Bicycling, 6 mph	160	240	312
Bicycling, 12 mph	270	410	534
Jumping rope	500	750	1,000

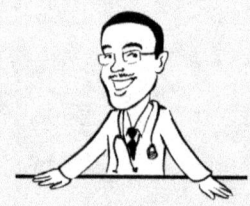

RANDY'S RULES

The Laborers' Health and Safety Fund of North America does the math on the relationship between physical activities and calories burned.
Please visit **www.lhsfna.org** for more information.

How to Count Calories

When trying to manage your weight, it's all about calories. Weight management is simple; to gain weight, eat more calories than you burn. To lose weight, eat fewer calories than you burn. To know what you are doing, keep count of your calories. Look at the number of calories per serving in the foods you are eating. Decide how much (how many servings) to eat, based on your daily calorie goals.

In general, a 2,000-calorie diet, upon which the FDA has based its labeling, is reasonable for most average-sized individuals who want to maintain weight and do little exercise. Exercising on a 2,000-calorie diet may help with weight loss. So, in regard to an individual food, a good rule of thumb is: 40 calories is a low-calorie food, 100 calories is moderate, and 500 calories is high for a particular food.

Frequently Asked Questions

The American Heart Association is an invaluable source of information and inspiration. The service it provides to America's families is hard to match. To take full advantage of its offerings, visit its website at www.americanheart.org. Here are some FAQs from its site that address some vital issues about calories.

1. What are discretionary calories?

You have a daily energy need—the calories your body needs to function and provide energy for your activities.

Think of it as a budget. You'd organize a real budget with "essentials" (rent and utilities) and "extras" (vacation and entertainment). In a daily calorie budget, the essentials are the minimum number of calories you need to meet your nutrient needs.

Select low-fat and no-sugar-added foods to make good "buys" with your budget. Depending on the foods you choose and the amount of physical activity you do each day, you may have more calories left over for extras that can be used on treats like solid fats, added sugars, and alcohol. These are discretionary calories, or calories to be spent at your discretion. A person's discretionary calorie budget varies depending on how physically active she is and how many calories she needs to consume to meet her daily nutrient requirements.

2. How are the remaining discretionary calories consumed if not as added sugars?

Discretionary calories are in addition to those that supply the nutrients to your body for daily function and activity. Your body does not actually need them to function. Common sources of discretionary calories are fats, oils, and alcohol. Discretionary calories can be used to eat foods that are high in fat or contain added sugars, to add fats or sweeteners to the lean versions of foods, and to eat or drink items that are mostly fat, sugar, or alcohol (candy, cake, beer, wine or soda).

3. Why are "liquid calories" and "solid calories" different?

Some studies suggest that drinking too many calories is even more likely to cause weight gain than calories from solid foods. It is suggested that liquid calories are not as satisfying as calories consumed from solid foods, so people tend to consume more fluid calories to compensate. As a result, reducing liquid caloric intake has a stronger effect on weight loss than reducing solid calories.

Drinking calorie-containing beverages is connected with overweight and obesity. People should carefully monitor the calories they drink and get enough water to maintain proper hydration every day.

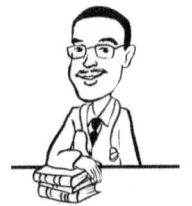

THE WRIGHT ADVICE

To really understand the relationship between how many calories you ingest and how many you expend doing various activities, check out the National Heart Lung and Blood Institute.

www.nhlbi.nih.gov/health/public/heart/obesity/wecan/healthy-weight-basics/balance.html

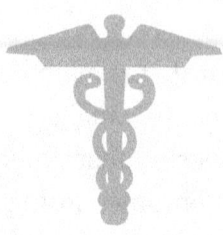

The Wright Reminders

Purchase a calculator.

Count your calories.

Figure out your excess calories.

Make a plan to change.

Exercise!

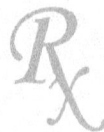

CHAPTER 10

Vitamins, Supplements, and Fads

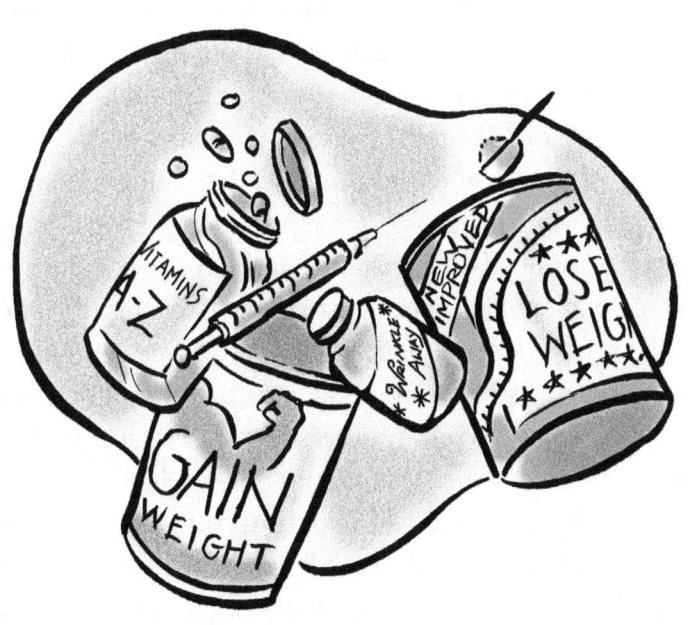

The Easy Fix

Our society thrives on immediate gratification and is obsessed with tangible, measurable results—in as short a time as possible. We all look for the easiest and most convenient ways to eat, get things done, and look super human. There's nothing wrong with convenience, living efficiently, and wanting to look better, but shortcuts are usually not as beneficial as they seem, especially when it comes to our bodies and our health.

People purchase vitamins and supplements for many different reasons. They fall prey to fads on a daily basis. Some are trying to compensate for poor eating habits; others are looking to receive perceived protective benefits against disease, and there's an unofficial club out there wishing to enhance any number of different performances by making themselves feel something more than merely better.

You have to admit, the thought of popping a pill and making all your ills disappear is very intriguing. We are constantly barraged by the vitamin and supplement industry, claiming that certain products are going to change the very definition of good health. Claims of this nature remind me of the alchemists of the 1800s who were trying to change basic metals into gold. They even sought to find the panacea which was a substance that would cure all ills.

Centuries later, we still cannot turn metal into gold, although many folks are still searching for the panacea. Now, giving alchemy its due credit, many of the methods used by those scientists actually gave birth to many techniques used in modern chemistry. When thinking of vitamins and supplements, it is important for us to put their use in proper perspective and not expect "metals to turn to gold."

Medical Myth #8
"If I take vitamins every day, who cares what I eat?"

Healthy individuals with access to a variety of foods do not normally need supplements. The American Heart Association feels that there is not enough data to suggest that supplements enhance or improve the human condition by replacing a fundamentally sound diet. The AHA specifically advises that vitamin supplements should not be used as replacements for a well-balanced diet.

The American Dietary Association recommends vitamins and/or dietary supplements only in specific cases, such as when a woman is pregnant or of child-bearing age, when a person has a daily caloric intake of less than 1,600 calories or a medical condition that limits food choices, such as a vegan or strict vegetarian diet, or if someone is elderly with a poor diet.

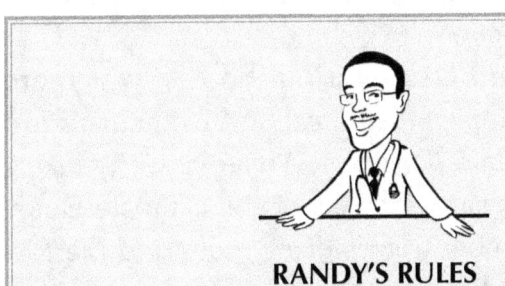

RANDY'S RULES
If you are at all unsure about taking a vitamin or supplement, consult your doctor.

We should not take the mindset that taking certain vitamins can replace eating fruits and vegetables. We should also be careful about looking for the panacea pill that cures all. In fact, some supplements have unknown side effects.

Save Your Money—and Your Life

I must smile and shrug whenever my patients ask me if they can take a pill to clean their colon, fight cancer, clear out their arteries, or cure their arthritis. As a religious man, I am not one to limit God, for He can do anything, but at this point in medical history, I know of no such pill and cannot even imagine one ever being created. We need to change our mindset from preferring a quick fix to doing the "Wright Thing," meaning taking care of our bodies the way God intended us to, eating the natural foods He gave us.

If that sounds too simple, then consider your car. You want it to run like a well-oiled machine, right? If I told you that a single liquid could be used as gas, windshield fluid, radiator fluid, and oil, would you believe me? Of course not! A car is far too complex for a single fluid to serve all these functions.

The same can be said for our bodies, which are infinitely more complex than a car. But we humans just can't seem to contain ourselves. We are always seeking the Holy Grail, or Fantastic Abs or the Ultimate Detox Diet. If you remember from *Indiana Jones and the Last Crusade*, the Holy Grail is not a shiny, fancy cup. It's a simple, modest vessel, inspiring inner beauty over outer appeal. So it is with our health. What Madison Avenue

Vitamins, Supplements, and Fads

and late-night infomercials advertise as sexy, quick-and-easy roads to ultimate health are quite likely to lead you to one frustrating dead end after the other.

The true road to a long and healthy life includes knowledge, moderation, and persistence. It begins with food, a necessary fuel for life, continues with exercise, also a necessity, and is punctuated by the need for a positive attitude. As we said earlier, if you don't have any special requirements and you eat how you are supposed to, then you don't need extra vitamins or supplements. The sad truth is, most Americans don't eat what they're supposed to—far from it—and they are prime candidates for vitamin and supplement manufacturers to prey on their insecurities and preferences for a quick-and-easy fix. It's almost as if the industry has been observing how Americans eat over the past few decades and came to realize that they could make a fortune offering vulnerable Americans a host of vitamins and supplements based on the fact that we don't want to bother watching what we eat so they can simply take care of that with a medley of pills, preservatives, and pipe dreams.

The same thing happens with getting enough sleep. Take this pill and you're off to dreamland. Groggy? Drink a ton of coffee and you'll go go go! Better still, try this energy drink! Want to lose weight? Pop a diet pill. Don't eat enough fruits and veggies? No problem, we've got your back. Who needs to eat real food when you can swallow greens in a bottle, fruit capsules, or protein shakes?

Time out. Let's give the vitamin and supplement industry a break. After all, there are many reputable companies, manufacturing quality products, and some people, especially those who don't eat a sufficiently well-balanced diet, can benefit from taking some of these products. For example, what about the ten-year-old child who won't eat anything green? No spinach, no broccoli, no salad greens—nothing! And this food aversion is not limited to green vegetables; it's any color vegetable, or fruit! None at all. Ever. Not once. Even when the pediatrician lays down the law, no dice!

That's when a vegetable pill can come to the rescue, so to speak, providing this child with a minimal amount of vegetable-based sources of vitamins and minerals. But while such a dosage is worthwhile, assuming the pill is all-natural, it can't be used as a substitute. Pills will never replace a good diet. They have appropriate uses, but far too many people use vitamins and supplements inappropriately, often out of sheer laziness.

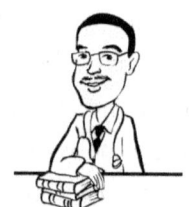

THE WRIGHT ADVICE

Before rushing off to purchase remedies you've seen advertised on television or in a magazine, think about what you are really trying to fix and is that the best way to do it?

Are those vitamins and/or supplements really necessary?

Or do you simply need to eat better, exercise, and get better quality sleep?

Vitamins, Supplements, and Fads

Vitamin	Function	Food Sources	Recommended Dietary Allowance (ages 25–50 years)
Vitamin A	Promotes growth and repair of body tissues, bone formation, healthy skin and hair. Essential for night vision, immune system integrity.	Liver, milk and dairy products fortified with vitamin A.	3,330 IU (men) 2,664 IU (women)
Beta-carotene (Converted to vitamin A in the body)	Serves as an antioxidant, may help protect against certain cancers, cataracts, heart disease.	Carrots, sweet potatoes, spinach, greens, pumpkin, apricots, watermelon, broccoli.	No RDA exists for beta-carotene.
Vitamin D	Aids in absorption of calcium, helps build bone mass and prevent bone loss. Helps maintain blood levels of calcium, phosphorus.	Sunlight, vitamin D-fortified dairy products, fish oils, tuna, salmon.	200 IU (ages 19–51) 400 IU (ages 51–70) 600 IU (age 70+)
Vitamin E	Helps protect cells from free radical injury. Serves as an antioxidant and may help protect against heart disease, cataracts, certain cancers. Needed for normal growth and development.	Nuts, seeds, wheat germ, margarine, vegetable oils, salad dressings made with vegetable oils.	14.9 IU (men) 11.92 IU (women)
Vitamin K	Necessary for normal blood clotting, bone health.	Green, leafy vegetables, liver.	80 mcg (men) 65 mcg (women)

Vitamin	Function	Food Sources	Recommended Dietary Allowance (ages 25–50 years)
Vitamin B Complex			
Thiamin (B1)	Essential for converting carbohydrates to energy. Needed for normal functioning of the nervous system and muscles, including heart muscle.	Pork, whole and enriched grains, dried beans and peas, brewer's yeast, sunflower seeds.	1.2 mg (men) 1.1 mg (women)
Riboflavin (B2)	Helps in red blood cell formation, nervous system functioning, and release of energy from foods. Needed for vision and may help protect against cataracts.	Liver, milk, yogurt, mushrooms, enriched grains, whole grains.	1.3 mg (men) 1.1 mg (women)
Niacin	Promotes release of energy from foods and proper nervous system functioning.	Enriched grains, whole grains, mushrooms, bran, tuna, salmon, chicken, beef, liver, peanuts.	16 mg (men) 14 mg (women)
Pyridoxine (B6)	Essential for protein metabolism, nervous system and immune function. Involved in synthesis of hormones and red blood cells.	Liver, tuna, beef, pork, spinach, bananas, soybeans, sunflower seeds.	Men: 1.3 mg (ages 19–50) 1.7 mg (ages 51+) Women: 1.3 mg (ages 19–50) 1.5 mg (ages 51+)
Folic acid	Needed for normal growth and development and red blood cell formation. Reduced risk of neural tube birth defects. May reduce risk of heart disease.	Green leafy vegetables, orange juice, organ meats, sprouts, sunflower seeds.	400 mcg

Vitamins, Supplements, and Fads

Vitamin	Function	Food Sources	Recommended Dietary Allowance (ages 25–50 years)
Vitamin B12	Vital for blood formation and healthy nervous system.	Animal organs, oysters, clams, eggs.	2.4 mcg
Biotin	Assists in metabolism of fatty acids and utilization of B vitamins.	Cheese, egg yolks, cauliflower, peanut butter, liver.	30 mcg
Pantothenic acid	Aids in normal growth and development.	Mushrooms, liver, broccoli, eggs. (Most foods contain some of this nutrient.)	5 mg
Vitamin C	Promotes healthy cell development, wound healing, resistance to infection. Serves as an antioxidant and may help protect against certain cancers, cataracts, and heart disease. Promotes iron absorption.	Citrus fruits, strawberries, cantaloupe, tomatoes, broccoli, mustard greens, cauliflower, green pepper, cabbage, asparagus, potatoes.	60 mg
Calcium	Essential for developing and maintaining healthy bones and teeth. Assists in blood clotting, muscle contraction, nerve transmission. Reduces risk of osteoporosis.	Dairy products, green, leafy vegetables, canned fish, tofu.	1,000 mg (ages 19–50) 1,200 mg (ages 51+)
Phosphorus	Works with calcium to develop and maintain strong bones and teeth. Enhances use of other nutrients. Essential for energy metabolism, DNA structure, and cell membranes.	Dairy products, meats, poultry, fish, eggs, whole grains, nuts and seeds, processed foods.	700 mg (age 19+)

Vitamin	Function	Food Sources	Recommended Dietary Allowance (ages 25–50 years)
Magnesium	Activates nearly 100 enzymes and helps nerves and muscles function.	Green vegetables, legumes, cereal, fish, whole bran.	Men: 420 mg (ages 31–70) Women: 320 mg (ages 31–70)
Sodium	Necessary for maintaining fluid balance. Transports nutrients across cell membranes.	Table salt, milk, processed meats (luncheon meats, ham, bacon), snack chips, crackers.	Not more than 2,400 to 3,000 mg
Potassium	Maintaining fluid balance.	Spinach, brussels sprouts, bananas, potatoes, tomatoes, orange juice, cantaloupe.	1,600 to 2,000 mg
Chloride	Necessary for maintaining normal acidity in the stomach. Helps carry carbon dioxide to the lungs.	Table salt.	750 mg
Iron	Needed for red blood cell formation and function.	Liver, meats, green leafy vegetables, enriched breads and cereals.	10 mg (men) 15 mg (women)
Zinc	Essential part of more than 100 enzymes involved in digestion, metabolism, reproduction and wound healing.	Meat, liver, poultry, fish, oysters, other seafood, whole grains, eggs.	15 mg (men) 12 mg (women)
Iodine	Helps regulate, growth, development, metabolism. Necessary for normal thyroid function.	Iodized salt, salt-water fish, dairy products, white bread.	150 mcg

Vitamins, Supplements, and Fads

Vitamin	Function	Food Sources	Recommended Dietary Allowance (ages 25–50 years)
Selenium	Necessary for normal growth, development, use of iodine in thyroid function. May reduce risk of certain cancers.	Whole grains, fish, seafood, liver, meats, eggs.	70 mcg (men) 55 mcg (women)
Copper	Involved in iron metabolism, nervous system function, bone health, synthesis of proteins. Plays a role in pigmentation of skin, hair, eyes.	Liver, seafood, nuts, seeds.	1.5 to 3.0 mg
Manganese	Necessary for normal development of skeletal and connective tissues. Involved in metabolism of carbohydrates.	Whole grains, cereals.	2.0 to 5.0 mg
Fluoride	Dental health, incorporation into bones and teeth.	Most plants and animals, fluoride-fortified toothpaste, some water supplies.	Men: 4 mg (ages 19+) Women: 3 mg (ages 19+)
Chromium	Normal glucose metabolism.	Egg yolks, whole grains, pork.	50 to 200 mg
Molybdenum	Needed for metabolism of DNA and RNA.	Milk, beans, breads, cereals.	75 to 250 mg

Source: United States Department of Agriculture

Natural Remedies

I get asked a lot about vitamins, supplements, and herbs. People are funny; for some reason we, as a society, are taking positions more and more against pharmaceutically made medications and prefer taking natural herbs instead. If taking a "natural" product means buying a special herb at a health food store that is also made by a for-profit company that may not be FDA regulated, it might not make any more sense than filling your doctor's prescriptions!

I'm not claiming that our giant pharmaceutical companies are harmless entities that should be blindly trusted. We know that they are for-profit companies that watch their bottom line, but don't we all? How many of you work for free? America is a profit-driven country, fueled by innovation, so let's not go off the deep end and mistrust an industry just because it makes money. After all, it also saves millions of lives. But those same people who distrust the pharmaceutical industry will also trust anyone who tells them that their juice or pill will cure cancer, heal heart disease, and make them younger.

Hold on. All those products that you buy without a prescription may not be FDA approved, meaning they probably have not been thoroughly tested for safety and effectiveness. In other words, I could make a pill tomorrow out of sugar (for taste) and caffeine (to give you a rush of energy), throw in some vitamin C (to claim nutritional value), and call it *Dr. Wright's Youth Pill*. I could hire a fancy marketing firm to promote my pill as a nutritional source of energy and do a few controlled surveys to prove that this product has value. If I'm lucky, I'll get a celebrity endorsement and have a parade!

This is a crude example, but it demonstrates that a miracle pill is not likely to satisfy your desire for a natural way to better health. There are some legitimately good nutritional supplement companies, and they do have a place in certain circumstances, but it is not the automatic answer for the majority of us.

STOP!

EXERCISE BREAK!

Time for your fave five times four.

Uh, that would be 20 minutes,
in case you're wondering.

Not to be showing off my math skills; it's just
that I want you to get active and do it now!

No supplement or vitamin can replace movement.

Supplements to Avoid

According to a recent report from the Food and Drug Administration, certain supplements, marketed by irresponsible manufacturers, can actually do much more harm than any possible good. We recommend you do diligent research before throwing away your money and risking your health by taking any of these: aconite, bitter orange, chaparral, colloidal silver, coltsfoot, comfrey, country mallow, germanium, greater celandine, kava, lobelia, and yohimbe.

In a September, 2010 release, *Consumer Reports* (www.ConsumerReportsHealth.org) did a great job of investigating and identifying these supplements, which have been linked by scientific evidence to cancer; coma; kidney, liver, and heart damage; and death. But most supplement manufacturers, in an industry with nearly $27 billion a year in profit, are going to do whatever they can to keep the cash flowing. As long as the FDA doesn't outlaw any of these supplements, they will continue to market them as "cures for what ails ya."

Just like the medicine men used to do back in the wild, wild West, salesmen today will do whatever it takes to make a buck. It's up to you to do your due diligence, through Internet research and connecting with your doctor.

What's Right for My Family and Me?

We make decisions about our family's health based on many factors, including cultural backgrounds, available knowledge, financial considerations, faith, and current trends in society. Choosing whether to use vitamins and/or supplements should be an educated decision influenced by consultation with your doctor. Ultimately, it's your decision, but do yourself and your family a favor by researching what interests you, and again, check with your family doctor about what might be best for each of you.

Vitamins, Supplements, and Fads

Ben Franklin and a lot of other wise people had it right. They were masters of the fundamentals. They ate well, exercised, and got adequate sleep each night. If we keep this big three going, we probably won't need many "extras."

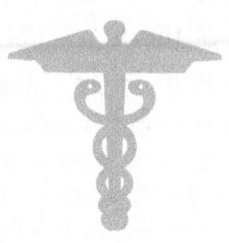

The Wright Reminders

Consult with your doctor about taking vitamins.

Research supplements before adding them to your diet.

Make sure that whatever pill you wish to take is approved by the FDA.

Assess and adjust your diet before settling for popping pills.

Exercise!

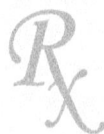

CHAPTER **11**

WATER BREAK!!!

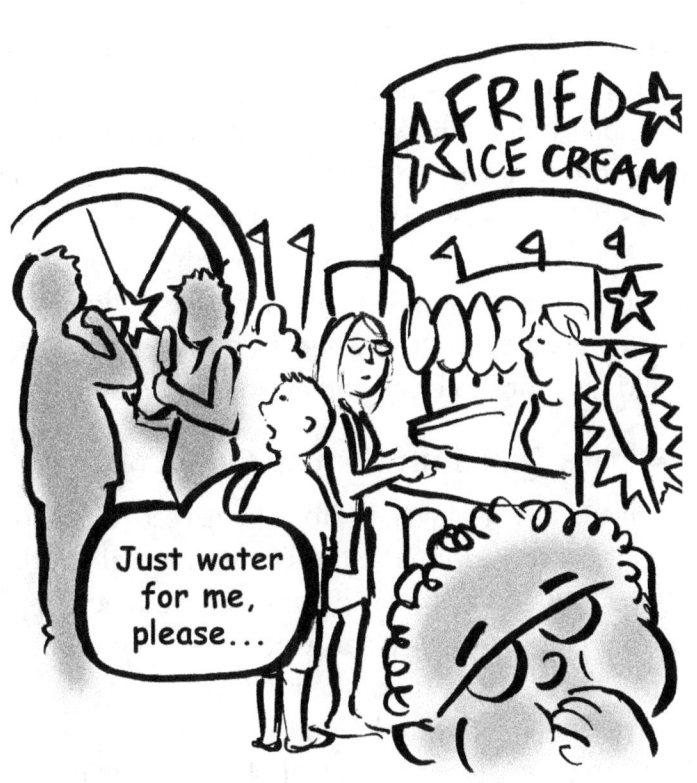

The Magic Elixir

Back in the day when charlatans and hucksters were peddling miracle cures at county fairs, they invariably tried passing off a bottle of water as a "tonic for what ails ya," a magic elixir and the key to a healthy life. They weren't entirely full of it because the water in those bottles really does hold one key to our well-being.

The average human body is composed of between 50 to 65 percent water, so it makes perfect sense that we pay close attention to maintaining that mix with a daily dose of good, clean H_2O. We humans are not the same as other species. We need the fresh stuff. But contrary to popular belief (and what the bottled water industry wants us to believe), we don't need to drink at least eight glasses of water every day. We get plenty of water from other sources—20 percent alone from the water content in food—so the best rule might simply be to drink when you are thirsty. Of course, when it's really hot you should remind your kids to drink and avoid dehydration.

What's That Stuff Coming Out of My Tap?

Tetrachloroethylene. Radium. Bromoform. Lead. Chloroform.

I'm sad to report that the Environmental Working Group (EWG), a national organization advocating for health related issues—clean water being chief among them—has detected more than 300 pollutants during a prolonged nationwide study conducted between 2004 and 2009, which included more than 47,000 drinking water utilities and 20 million test results. It discovered that more than 50 percent of the chemicals are still unregulated and considered legal, no matter how high their concentration might be.

(Wait a minute. Chloroform? Isn't that what they use as embalming fluid?)

The EWG rated my home, Houston, Texas, number 95 out of 100 American cities with the best and worst water utilities. The Texas Commission on Environmental Quality conducted the tests on the City of Houston Public Works, which serves approximately 2,700,000 people, and contributed them to EWG's national database. After conducting 22,083 tests in Houston, compared with the national average of 420 per municipality, it found 46 chemical pollutants, compared with the national average of 8 and 18 chemicals, which exceeded health guidelines, compared with 4 on average nationally.

For some reason, the Environmental Protection Agency has not reported any violations in Houston since 2004. Then again, it probably shouldn't come as any big surprise. Many government agencies throughout the world, charged with the responsibility of protecting its citizens, have failed to do an adequate job. When it comes to my family, I feel I should get as much information about the water we are drinking, bathing in, and using to water our growing vegetables in the backyard.

Perhaps I should move a couple of hundred miles to the north and settle in Arlington, Texas, which the EWG ranks number one as the top water utility system in the country. Between 2004 and 2008, while conducting 1,832 tests on a water system that serves approximately 290,000 people, it discovered only 15 chemical pollutants, compared with the national average of 8, and 7 chemicals, as opposed to 4, which exceeded health guidelines.

Providence, Rhode Island is rated number 2, Boston is 5, Las Vegas is down at 98, and San Diego isn't doing much better at 92.

Bottled or Bust

In 1974, Congress passed the Safe Drinking Water Act in order to regulate the nation's public drinking water supply and protect sources of drinking water. The U.S. Environmental Protection Agency (EPA), along with its state partners, administers these efforts. You can check the Consumer Confidence Report, which your local water supplier must mail to homeowners each year in July. Those of you renting homes can get a copy at your local library or online. The report lists the average, acceptable levels of various contaminants in your local water. If you decide to have your home waters tested, the EPA can help you. Go to www.epa.gov/safewater/faq/sco.html for a list of certified labs, or call your state health department.

There's no conclusive evidence that one type of water is purer than the other. Bottled water may be safer if your local tap water contains excessive levels of any contaminants. I would recommend doing your due diligence when it comes to your water supply and your health. After all, water is a main staple of our daily diet.

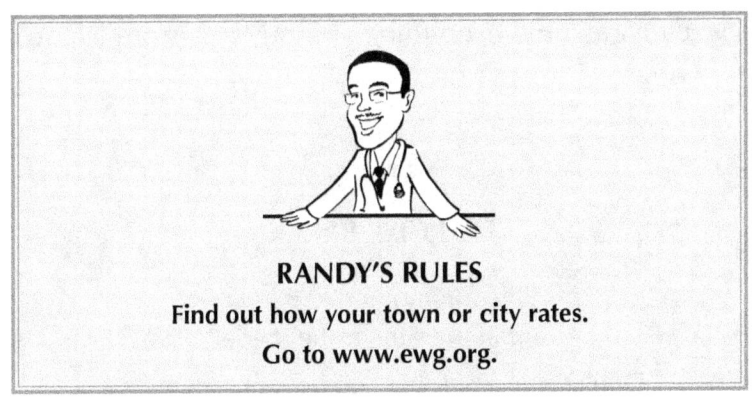

RANDY'S RULES
Find out how your town or city rates.
Go to www.ewg.org.

Medical Myth #9
***All bottled water must be safe. It has to be.
It comes in a bottle!***

You'd think so, right? But is it even logical to assume that all bottled water comes from a clean, fresh source? Wouldn't it be so easy to just fill up a million bottles of water, straight from the tap, slap a picture of a mountain stream around the bottle and call it "Nature's Gift" or something like that, and sell it to unsuspecting customers interested in avoiding the possible dangers of tap water? Actually, I'll bet some companies are already doing that and all of us have probably fallen prey to their effective advertising.

You simply don't have to do that. You can check the labels on bottled water and see where the water comes from. If it says that the water comes from an unnamed municipal source, it's glorified tap water. You can call the company and ask. You can check with the Better Business Bureau, the Environmental Protection Agency, or the Food and Drug Administration.

Don't assume everything you buy in a store is good for you.

> **STOP!**
> **EXERCISE BREAK!**
> It's time for another 20 minutes of fun in the sun (or the shade).
> Drink some water (tap, bottled, or otherwise) before, a bit during, and a little after.
> Staying hydrated is essential to good health.

Filters

It seems clearer and clearer that most tap and well water in the United States is nothing to really brag about. In fact, with industrial and environmental pollution on the rise, water is becoming less and less safe to bathe in, much less to drink. People are getting sick and don't often know why. Long-term illnesses and diseases can't always be traced back to the water sources, but research is pointing more and more to those possibilities. And, it's not only our rivers and streams that are producing these toxins. The plastic in some water bottles has been found to contain toxic chemicals, and in some cases the water itself was discovered to come from polluted sources.

Installing a quality water filtration system in your home can protect you from most of these risks. Reverse osmosis water purification systems can remove nearly all of the contaminants from city and well water. If you can't swing converting your entire home system, you can install water filters on individual sinks in your home. It's not only your kitchen sink that needs it. Installing a filter in your bathroom can also ensure better water quality for brushing your teeth and washing your face.

If installing filters poses problems, you can purchase water pitchers with filters that will significantly improve the quality of the water you are currently drinking. You can organize and deliver a healthy water supply in your home for you and your family. In fact, in some municipalities across the country, you may qualify for a subsidized filter system. Check with your local government agency or with your water utility company.

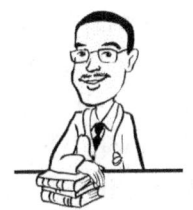

THE WRIGHT ADVICE

Using a water filter is usually cheaper than switching to bottled water.

The filter's instructions should specify which contaminates it can remove.

If you decide to go the bottled water route, choose a brand that includes fluoride.

The Beverage Wars

Water is the best liquid to provide our body with its fluid requirements; however, it's surely not the only drink that will suffice. We are inundated with beverage selections everywhere we turn. Fruit juices, yogurt drinks, vitamin water, power drinks, sodas—what an overwhelming mess of choices! Most of them are not good for you at all. Calorie and sugar content is off the wall with many of those choices. They are bad for your stomach, your teeth, and your wallet. It's just a big trifecta of pain. You complain that your pants don't fit; you need a cavity filled, and you've run out of money—again.

Why? You have so many good options, but once again, you go for the easy fix. Yes, I agree that you can get a refreshing drink that counts toward your water intake, but you can quickly pack on the calories with many of them, which can lead to weight gain and another one of those dreaded cavities. Last time I looked, dental insurance wasn't so easy to come by, and a visit to the dentist wasn't getting any cheaper. Also, consumption of soft drinks instead of more nutritious drinks, such as milk and water, can deprive you of valuable nutrients. If you must drink something sweet and fizzy, try to find a low-calorie drink version.

Water is the most important thing we can drink, and it's essential for our existence. Humans can go six or more weeks without eating, but we can survive only a few days without water. Water is found in essentially every part of our body and is involved in temperature regulation, digestion, lubrication, and structure. Without water, life as we know it would end.

According to the USDA, men 19 to 30 years old should drink 3.7 liters of water a day, and for women 19 to 30, it is 2.7 liters a day. As we have found out for many of us in the United States, it's probably best if we avoid drinking tap water, especially without a filtration system of some kind.

When we are on the run, be picky about the bottled water you choose to drink. In fact, why not carry a thermos of filtered water from home? You'll be sure it's clean and fresh and you'll save a great deal of money over the course of a year.

Let's stay on that for a second. If you're a person who is trying to drink a steady amount of water on a daily basis, you may drink a couple bottles of water each day while you're away from home. With the average cost being about one dollar per bottle, that's two dollars a day. If you use filtered water from home, you can save more than $700 per year!

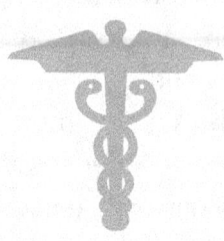

The Wright Reminders

Drink plenty of water.
(Cool water before a meal can reduce your appetite and may actually taste better, too.)

Research your local water supply.

Read water bottle labels before buying.

Choose water over juice and soda.

Use water filters at home.

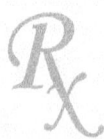

Part Three
Dr. Wright's Prescription for
Busy Families On The Go

CHAPTER 12

Home and Away: The Economics of Family Health

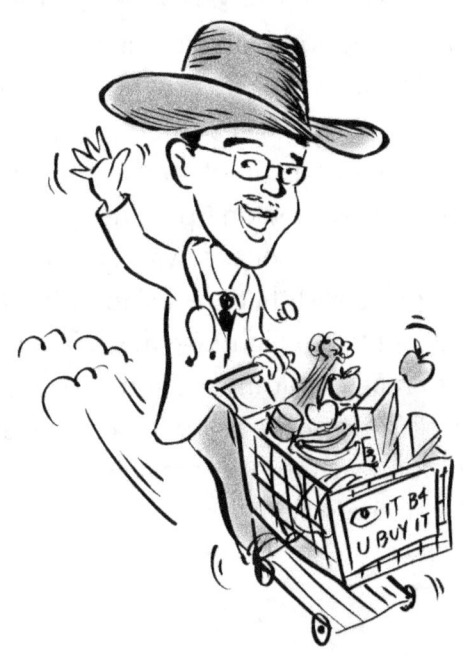

Are We Really What We Eat?

Yes we are, and the biggest problems with that is most of the time we don't really know what we're putting into our bodies. We don't have any idea if the food we buy is cost effective, especially when it comes to our health. Food, money, and health are very much related. Did you ever stop to consider the relationship between what you eat and how much you pay—or will pay in the future—for your health care?

First, let's consider what happens on a typical day. After gulping down some coffee on an empty stomach, we rush out of the house, undernourished and stressed. On our way to work, we're suddenly so hungry that we stop at a bagel shop to grab something to eat in the car. Twenty minutes later, stuck in traffic, we're sitting in a pile of crumbs from a bagel made of white flour, we've slogged down a second cup of coffee, and we're munching on that donut we couldn't pass up. Our next stop is at a convenience store because we have a stomachache from all the coffee and that giant slab of butter they put on the bagel. At the stoplight, we're straining to open up the antacid to relieve our indigestion and stop feeling so bloated. By the time we get to work, our system is out of whack, our blood sugar levels are all over the place, and we're shorter in the wallet.

All of this could have been prevented in just five extra minutes at home. We could have eaten any number of quick and simple foods, had a better quality drink, and taken a healthy snack with us into the car, in case we got hungry again during our commute. There's no need to spend money on a second cup of coffee, a bagel, a donut, and a bottle of antacid. There's even less need to have that stress you out for the rest of your day at work. Better health and keeping more money in our pockets come from a combination of common sense, thrift, and preventative care. Save your body and your bank account all at the same time.

If we take the long look at our future health, what will we feel like if we keep starting our days off harried and hungry for years on end? What will the cost be in terms of our wellness and our financial resources? Abuse like that will add up and take its toll. But it doesn't have to.

> "I want to start by taking a new approach that emphasizes prevention and wellness so that instead of just spending billions of dollars on costly treatments when people get sick, we're spending some of those dollars on the care they need to stay well."
>
> *President Barack Obama*
> *2009*

How to Read a Food Label

The first thing we need to do is know what we're eating, and that starts with reading food labels. You might say that food labels are our greatest allies in the quest for better health. Consider the example of Amanda and Kate shopping for milk. They are both in a hurry to get home after work and make dinner for their family. Amanda grabs a half-gallon of whatever is on sale and heads to the register. When she gets home, she realizes that her choice of milk was not so good; it's high in calories, full of fat, and has more cholesterol than anyone would recommend.

Kate goes to the exact same dairy section of the same store and takes about ten to twenty additional seconds to look at the food label on the side of the milk carton. Even though it costs 79 cents more, she selects the milk with fewer calories, 1% fat content, and a tolerable amount of cholesterol. Kate leaves the store less than a minute after Amanda.

Both Kate and Amanda want to satisfy the needs of their families, which means purchasing a product that is healthy and tastes good. Kate can have it both ways, and it takes her only a few extra seconds to know what she's purchasing.

Knowledge is power, and learning to read and understand the nutritional labels on foods will give you a whole new view of what you are feeding yourself and your family. This education will empower you to make better choices and save money. You're lucky. Twenty years ago, this information was not readily available.

In 1990, the Nutritional Labeling and Education Act (NLEA) was passed. This act mandated that all prepackaged food display a nutritional label. This gave consumers the ability to make more informed choices about the foods they eat. Learning to properly read and apply the information on a nutritional label is a powerful tool in our quest to lead a healthier life. So, let's take apart the label and learn what it's really telling us.

Those sandwich cookies look so good on the package! Of course they do. The cookie company was smart and hired an accomplished photographer or illustrator to make them look deliciously irresistible. You know deep down they're not so good for you, and your doctor told you to stay away from them, but they look so good on that shiny plastic wrapper and you just can't help it now, can ya? SOLD! And eventually eaten of course.

Now, if you had just taken a moment to read the label on the back of the package, it might've been a different story. Eye it before you buy it. In other words, read it and weep, because once you see what's in those cookies, you'll make the right choice.

Calculating the Numbers

Let's start by deciphering what's in the food you eat. In order to determine whether something is healthy, it's not only essential to know where the food comes from and how it's prepared. We need to know how much of it we should be eating.

Welcome to the world of Daily Value (DV) and the percent of Daily Value (%DV). The FDA has done us a big favor by determining limits on how much of a specific nutrient we should eat on any given day. The numbers are based on a 2,000 or 2,500-calorie diet (depending on your size and activity level). DV information is not food specific, but it does represent general eating goals.

Take a look at the sample label on the next page. It shows you just what you ought to be looking for. You'll see its intended serving size and the amount of servings in the container. Next, you'll see the amount of calories per serving, and how many of those calories come from a fat source. The largest section includes essential data on fats, cholesterol, sodium, fiber, sugars, and protein. That's followed by vitamin and mineral content.

All together, it takes just a few seconds to scan the label for what's bad for you and what's good for you, with any given food. Once you know the basics, which have been dished out throughout this book, you can make your shopping expedition a much more beneficial outing for you and your family.

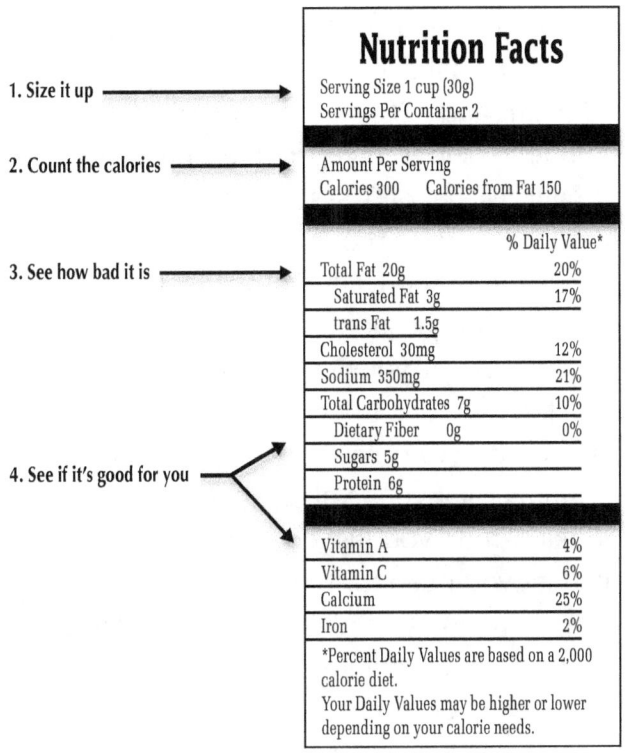

What the Labels Mean

Most food labels list nutritional values as follows:

Total Daily Calories		**2,000**	**2,500**
Total Fat	Less than	65g	80g
Sat Fat	Less than	20g	25g
Cholesterol	Less than	300mg	300mg
Sodium	Less than	2,400mg	2,400mg
Total Carbs		300g	375g
Dietary Fiber		25g	30g

The FDA recommends that if our goal is a 2,000-calorie diet, we should limit our daily intake of saturated fats to less than 20 grams and 300 grams of carbohydrates.

In order to help us compare individual food products, the FDA utilizes the %DV system. The %DV is determined for an individual food product, and the %DV represents the percentage of the Daily Value that product contains of the nutrient in question.

For example, if your favorite box of cookies has a saturated fat %DV of 23 per serving, and a serving is one cookie, then every cookie you eat gives you 23 percent of the saturated fat you're allowed for the day. If you eat four cookies, then you just consumed 92 percent of the saturated fat you need for the whole day!

Translation? You shouldn't eat those sandwich cookies. They're too high in saturated fat! Okay, you can eat one, since you love them so much, but then you will have to adjust your fat intake with everything else you eat that day.

The %DV may also help you decide what foods you need to eat more of each day. When it comes to fiber, most of us need to increase our intake. The FDA recommends at least 25 grams a day for a 2,000-calorie diet. When considering food choices, you want to look for foods with a high %DV, because that will help you reach your goal faster.

A quick and easy rule of thumb for using the %DV is as follows: 5%DV or less is low; 20%DV or greater is high. Food that contain 20%DV or higher of fat is too high. Food that contain 5%DV of fat or lower is preferred.

Solving the Mystery of What's in Our Food

If you're finding all these percentages and formulas confusing, here is how to make the information on food labels easier to decipher and ultimately more meaningful.

Remember: Read the labels first! Eye it before you buy it—because if you didn't realize it by now, you really can't judge a book (or packaged food) by its cover. For all the non-packaged foods you're purchasing—fruits, veggies, meats, fish, etc.—check out the website www.foodpyramid.gov for nutritional information.

Size It Up

The first rule of healthy eating is to know how much you are ingesting! We will discuss more in later chapters about portion size, but when it comes to reading labels, you need to first look at the serving size of the item you are about to buy and/or eat.

For example, you have kids; therefore you have ketchup. Look at the label. How much sugar is in there? One popular brand has four grams of sugar in one tablespoon–sized serving. If your kids are anything like mine, they probably suck up at least 10 tablespoons at many meals, both at home and in restaurants. That's 40 grams of sugar! And close to a thousand milligrams of sodium! The organic versions of this ketchup offer the same scary math. The difference is, the tomatoes and other ingredients are organic (and probably healthier), but the sugar and sodium content is as bad as the first ketchup! Once again, dosage is everything.

For the casual shopper, serving size can be the first trap that can lead to excessive eating. The information on the nutritional label is based on one serving size. You need to consider the serving size and the number of servings per package. If you are drinking a 12-ounce soda, and the listed serving size is 6 ounces (meaning there are two servings in the soda bottle), then you have to double all the values.

So if the label reads 60 calories per serving, and you drink the whole bottle, then you actually consumed 120 calories!

This can sometimes be tricky (I dare say deceptive), because most people assume that when they see the number of calories per serving, it means for the whole bottle (or package). When that occurs, and they fail to look at the serving size, they invariably tend to overeat.

Follow the golden rule with food labels. Always size up your food!

Count Your Calories!

Weight management in principle is simple; to gain weight, eat more calories than you burn. Conversely, to lose weight, eat fewer calories than you burn. To keep track of what's right for your situation you need to start counting calories. To do this, always look at the number of calories per serving in the food you are about to eat. Then decide how much (how many servings) you will eat based on your daily caloric goals. The FDA has determined that a 2,000-calorie diet is a reasonable goal for most average-sized individuals, who want to maintain weight and do little exercise. Therefore, exercising on a 2,000-calorie diet may help with weight loss.

In regard to any individual food, a good rule of thumb is:
- 40 calories is a low calorie food.
- 100 calories is a moderate amount of calories.
- 500 calories is high for a particular food.

See How Bad It Is

It's essential to evaluate the amount and types of fat contained in the foods you eat. We have learned that all fats are not bad, and our bodies actually need fat to survive. We also know that saturated fats and trans fats are two types of fats that we should avoid. For this reason, the FDA has mandated that they be listed separately. That should help you limit the amounts of bad fat that you eat.

Remember our rule of thumb: 5%DV or less is low and 20% or greater is high, so definitely avoid anything with 20%DV or more of fat.

See How Good It Is

As you advance on your pathway to healthier living, you will transition from just avoiding certain foods to looking for foods that enhance your eating plan. For example, you should maximize your intake of calcium, fiber, and a variety of vitamins, as recommended by your doctor and the FDA. Eating adequate amounts of these nutrients have been linked to a decrease in certain diseases, such as osteoporosis.

For more information on reading and using nutrition labels we recommend:

www.fda.gov/food/labelingnutrition/consumerinformation

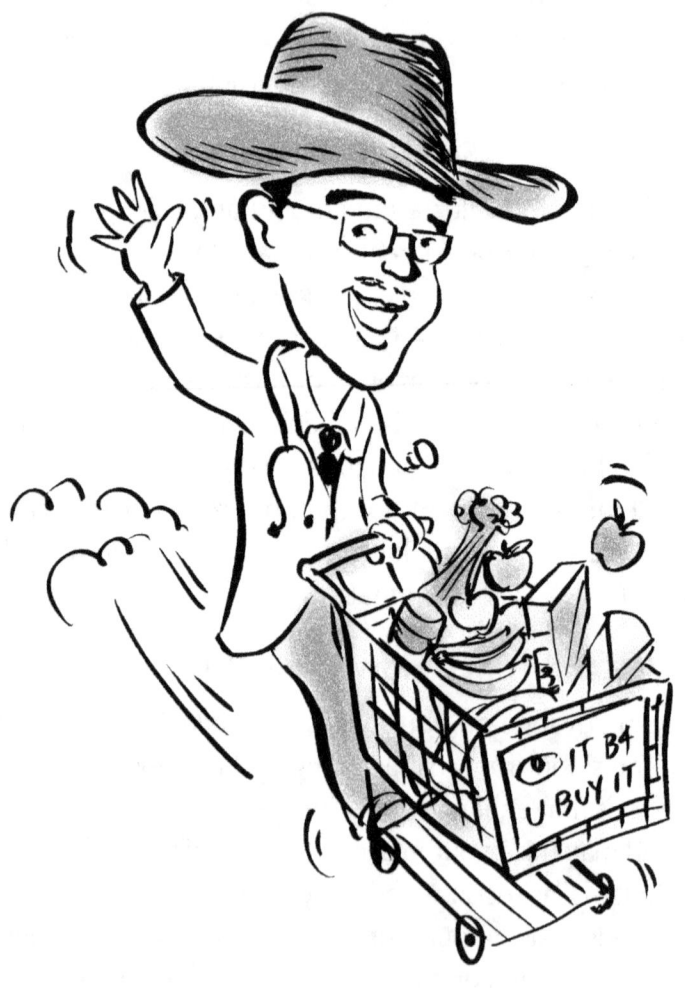

👁 IT B4 U BUY IT

If you live outside of Texas you may choose to leave your cowboy hat at home when going food shopping. But you'll be much better off if you remember my pet phrase, as seen on my shopping cart. For those not yet living in the Twitter age (which was me until about a week ago), it says "eye it before you buy it." Next time you're in a supermarket, overwhelmed with choices and not sure what's best for you and your family, read those labels carefully!

What's in Your Refrigerator?

Putting your new knowledge into practice is the best way to reinforce it. Let's do this by looking at what you have in your kitchen right now. Please remove three food items from your frig and place them on the counter for inspection.

Imagine we have a container of milk, a package of sliced lunchmeat, and a bottle of salad dressing. Let's analyze them, one by one, starting with 2% reduced fat milk.

Your average glass—a one cup serving of 244 grams—contains 122 calories (43 of them from fat) with 3.1 grams of saturated fat, 20 milligrams of cholesterol, 8.1 grams of protein, and 12.3 grams of sugar. While a glass of milk does provide a nice dose of Vitamin D, riboflavin, Vitamin B12, calcium, and phosphorus, that doesn't rank it terribly high on the general health meter. Its rating drops because of the high content of saturated fats and all the calories it offers from sugar.

Solution: fat-free skim milk.

That lunchmeat (turkey breast meat) is worse. Take an average portion of ham that you'd include in a sandwich on a normal day. One serving has 30 milligrams of cholesterol, more than 10 grams of protein, and 849 milligrams of sodium. The good news is that ham can be fairly low in fat and sugar and high in phosphorus and zinc. The bad news is how it boosts your cholesterol count and explodes your sodium meter.

Solution: low-sodium, low-fat packages of meat. As Rafiki says in *The Lion King*, "Look haaaarder." You can find healthy alternatives.

It gets even more discouraging when we consider the typical Italian salad dressing you've got chilling. Ouch. You might think a simple, little condiment would be harmless, but be warned. Commercial salad dressings are potent, and most people pay no attention when dosing their salads with dressing.

"I'm eating salad. Okay?" your best friend says, as you watch her douse her bowl with dressing.

"Good choice, but watch the dressing," you reply, trying not to gag.

"Give me a break!" she says. *"I can pour on as much dressing as I want if I'm eating salad! Right?"*

Pause. So as not to jeopardize your friendship, you consider your response.

I feel sad because I've heard that rationale way too often. Here's the unfortunate truth about one of the most basic foods we carelessly eat when we think we're dining well. Most of the trouble comes from portion control. The serving size on nearly all salad dressings is two tablespoons. How I wish we used only that much! Next time you're in a restaurant, watch how most people pour dressing over their salads. Two innocent tablespoons quickly becomes three or four times that amount. If an average salad dressing has one to two grams of fat, you've actually slathered at least six or seven grams of fat on your "healthy" salad. If two tablespoons contains more than 500 grams of sodium, you've probably added over 2,000 grams to your salad in one fell swoop.

Conclusion? You have choices! Don't forget that you control what you put in your body and in the twenty-first century, here in America, you have almost unlimited options when it comes to finding healthy foods. It's up to you how you control your dosage.

A Pantry Makeover

Let's take everything we've learned about food labels and start fixing things at home. No matter where you store your food, it's a good idea to examine each item, see if it makes sense to keep, and consider whether you may want to eliminate it or simply replace it with something better. When trying to create healthy eating habits, anything you can do to tip the odds in your favor will ultimately prove hugely advantageous.

Here is a little secret: if it's not in your pantry, you won't be able to eat it at midnight when nobody is watching and the temptation is greatest! How do you pull that off? Simple. Don't bring food into your home that you and your family really shouldn't eat. In order to remove the guesswork and the anxiety of choosing what to have in your pantry just follow the suggestions in this chapter. You'll end up making your pantry family-friendly, protecting you (and whoever else may be prowling the kitchen) from getting into too much trouble when those midnight cravings sound their alarm.

You can do this several ways, depending on your personality and your family's quirks. You can do the proverbial "Shock and Awe" by completely restocking your pantry in one aggressive and awe-inspiring sweep, together with your kids. Or you can pick a single category, say snacks, and clean up that section first. The next week you can revise your pasta and rice supply, and so on. Or you can simply look at the list provided here and slowly transition certain items over time.

Personally, I recommend the total Shock and Awe approach. Any food you choose to remove from your home can be brought to a shelter that will be happy to make use of any unopened food it can collect. If that technique is too overwhelming, try a complete makeover, one category at a time. Doing either of these will give you a strong sense of accomplishment. It will also help you to quickly get rid of the foods in your home that are not in your best interest.

Since you're reading this book, it's probably safe to assume that you want to start this process and get things done. So let's think big and go with the Shock and Awe method, with you making whatever modifications you may need to satisfy your style.

First, gather your family together and ask them to remove everything from your pantry, making piles of similar products on the kitchen table (rice, pasta, snacks, etc.). Examine what's there and identify all the foods that you should avoid or eliminate. Once you do that, follow the list of foods to add to your pantry and prepare to go shopping!

Foods to Eliminate from Your Pantry

1. High sugar and high-calorie foods (cookies, breakfast cereals, snack bars).
2. Foods with trans fats, including: packaged foods (cake and baking mixes, some soups, cookies, candy, cakes and donuts, salad dressings [that are not fat-free]).
3. Highly processed foods that do little more than tickle your taste buds. Examples include mac and cheese mix, breakfast bars, many cold cereals, and white bread.
4. High-salt foods. Try using foods with low salt or no salt at all.

TIPS

1. Replace bakery mixes with flour, baking powder, and other products you'll need to bake from scratch (a great activity to share with your kids).

2. While you may not eliminate foods with trans fats (and saturated fats) entirely, you can start buying lower fat and lower calorie snacks, and you can purchase fewer of them, too. If they are not in the house, you can't eat them.
3. Try fruit.
4. If you must eat pretzels, try brands with low salt.
5. Be careful of deceptive "healthy" marketing. Some brands may claim to have included nutrients such as iron, folate, or vitamins, but what about the the rest of the ingredients? READ THE LABEL!

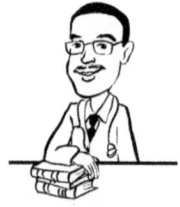

THE WRIGHT ADVICE

If it's creamy, crispy, or crunchy, and God didn't make it that way in the first place, then don't eat it!

Foods to Add to Your Pantry

1. Whole-wheat breads.
2. Whole-wheat pastas.
3. Whole-wheat anything—really!

4. Dry beans (black beans, black-eyed peas, lentils, kidney, lima, to name a few).
5. Whole grains (mother grains) in place of white rice, such as quinoa (see cooking instructions in Chapter 13) buckwheat, millet, amaranth, whole rye, corn, kamut, spelt, or even barley.
6. Brown rice. Make it your best friend.

> **A Word of Thanks to Anne Dubner,**
> Nutritionist and Dietitian extraordinaire,
> who has advised us throughout this book.
> Look for my interview with Anne in the next chapter.

Because being a good steward means not being wasteful, we suggest donating the food you don't want to a local food bank. Let them decide how best to use it. There are probably people in your city who are literally starving. In that situation, some food, even if it's not the healthiest choice, is better than no food at all. This is an opportunity for you to teach your children the value of good citizenship in their community and show them how to help those in need. In Chapter 15, we'll discuss further how you can affect your community with a plan for good health.

And now, here is the information you have been waiting for to redo your pantry and make your home healthier!

A New and Revised Shopping List for Your Pantry

Cereals / Breads / Grains:
    100% Whole-wheat bagels, breads, pita, and tortillas
    Brown rice
    Low-fat granola and unsweetened, low-fat, dry cereals
    Quinoa, millet, buckwheat, barley, or other whole grains (instead of rice)

Proteins:
    Beans, dry or canned without added fat
    Lentils
    Canned tuna, salmon, sardines (packed in water, low salt)
    Dry-roasted almonds, pecans, walnuts

Soups:
    Low-salt, low-fat soups (read the labels) and chilies
    Non-fat dressings

Snacks / Desserts:
    Popcorn, low-fat, low-salt
    Dried fruit
    Rice, corn cakes
    Low-fat oatmeal cookies
    Unsalted whole-wheat pretzels

Are You Really Hungry?

It's all fine and good to revamp your home food supply, but equally important is revising your family's mindset on eating, specifically how much. When restocking your pantry together, take the time to discuss what better eating choices really mean, and ask each and every member of your family to pay better attention, not only to what he eats, but to how much he is eating. Just because your pantry will now be full of better foods doesn't mean that's an excuse to consume them too fast!

STOP!

EXERCISE BREAK!

After you finish fixing up your pantry,
take 25 and get moving!

(What? Did they sneak in another five minutes?)

Remember the American Heart Association and their recommendation for a minimum of 30 minutes each day?

Okay. Your turn. Put down the book. Get moving!

Smart Shopping

First of all, stay on the perimeter of the store as much as possible. Every store, especially the bigger chains, wants to lure you into the aisles to buy food you don't necessarily need. Hey, if you don't go near it, it won't end up in your basket.

"But Dr. Wright," you protest so charmingly. "I'm going shopping in order to buy food for my family! How am I supposed to get everything I need by pushing my cart around the edges of the store and not going up and down every single aisle?"

Okay, let's start with what you do at home before you get to the store—your shopping list, the one thing that can save you time, grief, and money—and not necessarily in that order. It may take you five minutes to compose a list at home but that can save you much, much more once you get into the middle of the store. You can end up feeling bad simply because you can't remember what you need, or your kid is lobbying you for stuff you swore to yourself you wouldn't buy. Or worse still, you were a little hungry when you left home (your child was, too), and everything in the store is fast becoming attractive and too much of it is ending up in your shopping cart.

You could avoid all three of those curses by making a list beforehand at home. You can also avoid unnecessary purchases and crabby kids by giving everyone something to eat *before* you go shopping. Grocery store environments, with their warm lighting, attractive flooring, soft music, etc., are created to make you feel at home so you will want to stay longer and spend more money. Beware of free tasting, because most people who sample foods (especially when they are hungry) are likely to buy whatever it is the store is hawking. If you can't resist, at least make sure the foods you taste are on your list! When cruising the cereal aisle, for example, many grocery stores will shelve the popular kids' cereals at an eye level equal to where a child sits in a shopping cart. Avoid most of the items in this area. You will probably find the healthier cereals above or below this section.

Now, back to the store's perimeter. Start there to buy fresh fruits and vegetables. Choose produce that is ripe, firm, and unblemished. Don't be afraid to hold those clear cartons of berries up in the air and shake them a little to make sure there is no mold or pressure blemishes (from being packed tightly). Don't buy the big cartons of fruits; fruit typically does not last long. To avoid having spoiled fruit in your fridge, you may need to buy just enough to last you four or five days. If you can't get to the grocery store on a weekly basis and you need your fruits and veggies to last a little longer, try frozen alternatives. Frozen foods are just fine and are much better than canned foods, which tend to have higher salt contents.

Remember, one of your goals is to nourish your body with good nutrients, and fruits and vegetables are excellent sources. They are high in vitamins, fiber, and minerals but are low in calories! Stock up, because you should eat at least four to five servings of each of them every day. You should rotate the fruit and veggies you eat, to provide your body with a wide array of nutrients. Be adventurous. Try new types. You will be surprised how great these foods can taste and how great your body will feel after eating them!

As you continue circling the perimeter, you will most likely enter the bakery department. Oh, the smell of freshly baked bread will most definitely tickle your tummy! Enjoy the experience, but don't be tempted to buy what's not on your list. This section needs your 100 percent commitment to buying 100 percent whole grain products.

You may have grown up eating white bread, but the dirt you ate as a toddler may have offered you more nutritional value. Go whole grain. If the taste is too different at first, start with a small loaf and introduce it slowly into your routine. Over time, you will acquire a taste for it. Remember, one of your main goals is to minimize your intake of nutrient-poor food (white bread), and maximize the amount of nutrients you eat (whole-grain foods).

Back to your cart, moving swiftly through the supermarket.

The most exciting area tends to be the fresh meats section, with people yelling out tempting orders, such as "five pounds of bone-in steak, please" or "I'll take a dozen baby-back ribs," while the in-store chef is serving up samples of fresh, catfish filets! Step back, get a grip, and look intently at your list.

Fish is a great source of healthy, omega-3 fatty acids. The American Heart Association suggests that fatty fish (such as salmon, trout, or herring) should be eaten at least twice a week. When choosing meats, the AHA suggests that you buy lean cuts without the skin. The "loin" or "round" cuts of red meat and pork usually have lower fat contents. When you prepare them to eat, remember to remove any visible fat before you start cooking. When buying poultry, try to buy skinless white meat.

Home and Away: The Economics of Family Health

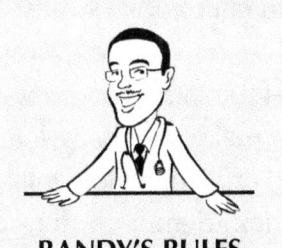

RANDY'S RULES
When cooking meats, make sure you grill, bake, or broil.
Stay away from frying!

Back to shopping and resisting the urge to purchase what you really don't need.

Typically, the lunchmeat section is next to the fresh meat counter. I would love to yell, "Run for your lives!" to get you out of this section, but I know, little Johnny needs food for lunch tomorrow. Hmmm. If we must satisfy this habit, then it's essential you read food labels. Most processed meats are high in saturated fat and salt, and should be avoided. Turkey products are good options, so pick the ones with the lowest fat and salt content. (Check the lunchbox recipes in Chapter 13 for some fun ideas.)

Moving along the perimeter, we will soon get to the dairy section. The rule here is simple: fat is bad, so don't buy it. Go for the fat-free milk, skim milk, or at the most, 1% milk.

For all the positive press milk receives (much of it through its own ad campaign), it is very much misused. For example, it seems more and more clear that whole milk contributes to childhood obesity! As your baby gets older, she should be transitioned away from whole milk to non-fat or low-fat milk. Speak to your pediatrician for the proper time to make the change. But as an adult, you should try to avoid drinking whole milk (especially in your morning lattes, drink them with non-fat or skim milk). If you are stuck on whole milk, then transition to milk with lower fat content because the change may save your life. Use the same principle with yogurts and cheeses; try to get the lowest fat content. In most stores you will find these alternatives, so it's really up to you to make good choices. No excuses!

When buying butter, which is likely to be near the milk, another simple tip is if the butter is solid at room temperature, don't eat it. Margarines or shortenings that are solid at room temperature are filled with harmful trans fats, so they should be avoided. Once again, reading the labels will help you navigate this tricky area. For cooking oils, use cold-pressed olive oils or liquid vegetable oils. You can even buy healthy oil sprays for cooking.

If you feel the urge to indulge in some treats, create limits! Each time you shop, pick one item that is totally frivolous but delicious. You can do that for yourself, and for each of your kids. Remember, libraries are for browsing. Grocery stores are for buying the things on your list and getting home as soon as possible.

Rethinking Household Products

While you're at the grocery store, tour the household section where cleaning supplies are sold and consider purchasing laundry detergent without dyes (biodegradable and hypoallergenic), dishwashing liquid and powders free of chemical additives, and cleaning supplies made from natural ingredients. These products may each cost a bit more, but in concentrated amounts they last longer and their long-term health benefits may be well worth the extra money.

Comparative Shopping

According to a recent survey conducted by the American Farm Bureau, "The average price for a half-gallon of regular whole milk was $2.00, up one cent from the prior quarter. The average price for a half-gallon of organic milk was $3.66, up nine cents from the fourth quarter of 2009 and eighty percent more expensive than regular milk. Compared to the first three months of 2009, a half-gallon of regular milk is eight percent cheaper and organic milk is one percent cheaper."

It can be a tough choice. Regular milk is known to be full of pesticides, hormones, antibiotics, and preservatives, all of which can compromise our immune systems and eventually breed infection. Long-term consumption of these foods has not been studied on a large scale, but common sense would tell anyone that it's better not to put that junk into our bodies. While it may be a stretch to purchase more expensive products, like organic milk, it may prove to be much cheaper in the long run, considering how much it costs these days to visit your medical practitioner. There's really no debate that organic milk is better than regular milk. If at all possible, we advise you to purchase milk and other dairy products that are organic or at least grown locally by health conscious farmers.

We suggest low-fat or non-fat organic products. Just because the fat in regular organic milk is organic, it's still fat, and that's a great big no-no.

The Truth About Organic Food

Okay, what's the big deal with organic food? Why should I risk going bankrupt buying these products for my family? What is it, really, and why is it so valuable? First of all, you won't end up in the poorhouse, but you will give yourself the chance to be healthier.

Maybe this litmus test will help to convince you.

> **Q:** What's in an eight-ounce "cocktail" of commercial milk?
> **A:** Milk, antibiotics, hormones, preservatives, and pesticides.
>
> **Q:** What's in an eight-ounce glass of organic milk?
> **A:** Milk.

The same can be said for most other foods. Traditional, commercially produced foods are compromised because of the very process that makes them cheaper than organic foods in the first place. To make a long story short—you get what you pay for!

Natural versus Organic

As the benefits of organic foods become more known and their popularity increases, food manufacturers are jumping on the bandwagon whenever possible. One of the silliest ways they are doing this is by touting their foods as "natural." Now, who would want to feed their family anything other than natural foods? So why are they pushing that word on us? Well, if you consider all of the foods made from man-made ingredients, it comes as no surprise that manufacturers are trying to lure us into buying things natural.

Imagine you are in the produce section and you pick up a traditionally grown apple. Next to it sits its organically grown counterpart. You hold one in each hand. They look pretty much the same. What's the difference, besides the price and the fact that the traditionally grown "natural" apple looks a bit shinier? It's all in what you don't see in the store.

The traditional apple grower uses chemical fertilizers to assist growth. They spray insecticides to reduce pests and disease, as well as chemical herbicides to manage weeds. Organic farmers, on the other hand, use natural fertilizers, such as manure or compost; avoid insecticides and herbicides; rotate crops; hand weed, or utilize mulch to conquer weeds.

As far as natural vs. organic goes, only foods with the "USDA Organic" label are authentic. Anything else is just a stab at getting you to fall for a fad, in this case, the relatively recent wave of popularity surrounding more healthy foods. While we're the first ones to advocate for healthier diets, we'd like you to pay attention to what's real and what's a second-rate imitation. Be a smart shopper!

> **FYI**
>
> The President's Cancer Panel (part of the National Cancer Institute) suggests you can reduce the risk of cancer by selecting foods that are free of pesticides, chemical fertilizers, antibiotics, or growth hormones. For more information, please visit deainfo.nci.nih.gov.

The Value of Buying Local

Locally grown food products, including fruits, vegetables, dairy items, baked goods, and even grass-fed beef, account for about one percent of all the food purchased in our country, according to a new report from the USDA's Economic Research Service (ERS). Food that goes directly from the grower to the buyer, in places such as farmer's markets, farm stands, etc., totaled about $1.2 billion in sales for 2007, less than half of one percent of the total food economy. That sounds tiny, but it's twice as much as it was ten years earlier. In fact, locally grown food is an industry growing much faster than commercially produced food. A huge increase in local farmer's markets is one of the biggest reasons.

What the USDA calls "direct-to-retail" sales by farms to institutions, including hospitals and schools, is currently nearing $10 billion in yearly sales. The USDA has much more information available on its website, featuring local food programs aligned with the 2008 Food and Farm Act.

In this day and age of chain stores and homogenous living, it's a welcome sight to see local, independently owned food vendors selling their wares. Supporting them is not only good for the environment and your community, oftentimes, the food they offer is tastier, better made (and grown), and healthier. There's nothing like the homemade touch!

Grass Fed or Processed?

Much like the debate over natural vs. organic, more and more people are learning about the benefits of grass-fed milk and meats. It's common sense. Cows that eat only grass and feed on unprocessed grains are probably healthier than their cousins, crammed inside stables, eating a steady diet of processed grain. Grass-fed cows produce meat with lower fat content, higher levels of heart-healthy omega-3 fatty acids, and more linoleic acid, which is thought to reduce heart disease and certain cancer risks.

We are not advocating adding meat to your diet, but when you do buy meat, it may be wise to consider purchasing grass-fed beef whenever possible.

Surviving Restaurants

You've cleaned your refrigerator. Examined your food labels. Navigated the grocery store. Investigated organic foods. You've fixed up your pantry. You're exhausted. You decide to take your family out for dinner. But have you opened up a new can of worms? Imagine this scene:

"Mommy, Mommy, can I have a cheeseburger and French fries and can I have extra fries and a milkshake and a Coke?"

"Daddy, I want ice cream, and then I want macaroni and cheese and French fries with chocolate syrup and extra butter and onion rings!"

"Yeah, I want onion rings, too!"

Even in the midst of being assaulted by your lovable, hungry children, watching your spouse shaking her head in mock horror at the amount of fat and starch your children want to immediately ingest, you can't help but notice all the enticing smells and the beautiful photographs on the menu, and you're secretly thinking, "I want everything!"

But you know better. Don't you? Your kids are excited to be out of the house, breaking up the routine, and you want to indulge them. You may even be thinking, I need to eat more because it's cheaper. STOP! Get a grip. The Happy Meal will make the inside of your child very UNhappy. The all-you-can-eat buffet shouldn't be taken literally. It's not a contest to actually find out how much food you can stuff inside yourself, all for the price of a single dinner. Look at the price your body will pay for doing something like that. While we're at it, pay attention to what some restaurants are offering at the salad bars. Just because you can fill your plate with everything they offer for one nice price, ask yourself if you really want to fill up on iceberg lettuce, hard-boiled eggs, and buckets of salad dressing. If you don't see it, you can ask for fresh spinach, sprouts, and dressing on the side. There's nothing sillier (or sadder) than watching someone at a salad bar, thinking she's eating well as she loads her plate with all kinds of fatty foods and high-calorie items, with so much dressing on top that you can barely see the food underneath.

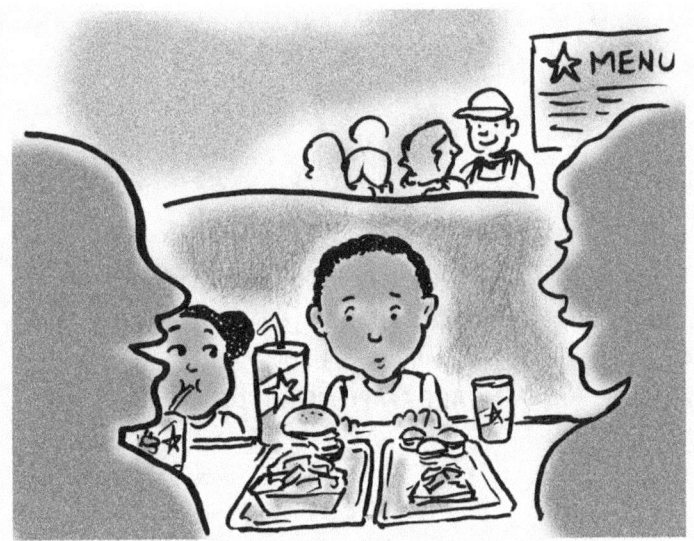

What's a boy to choose?
It's easy if he's offered only the healthy option.

Becoming a "Well Fed" Restaurant Guest

For those of you who teach their children at home to clean their plates you may want to reconsider that practice when you eat together in a family restaurant because when you consider the size of the portions many of these establishments serve, you will see that they are often way too much for any one child to eat during one sitting.

For those of you who are lucky enough to eat in high-end, fancy restaurants, please don't assume that just because you're eating expensive food that it's healthy for you. Speaking of fancy restaurants, one more thing: don't be afraid of foods you can't pronounce. Ask!

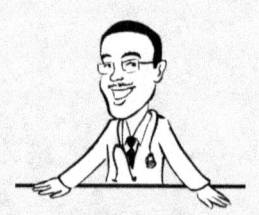

RANDY'S RULES
Keep your sauce on the side and your glaze nice and light.
It's your body.
TAKE RESPONSIBILITY!

ChefSpeak

Mark Holley, a famous chef in the Houston area, says that most chefs probably don't choose ingredients based on health alone, because they focus more on taste and appearance.

Home and Away: The Economics of Family Health

"We are all about coating your stomach with memories," says Mark, and if you've ever eaten at one of his restaurants, you'll agree. But even Mark admits some of his delicacies may not be terrifically healthy.

"Nobody trusts a skinny chef," Mark adds, "but we all need to redefine that. I can diet easier than anyone because I have all the resources I need in my kitchen, right here at work. I have the best food options at my disposal so I have no excuse for not eating well. It's about time many of us chefs and cooks start taking better care of ourselves and learning how to cook in more healthy ways for our clients."

You'll learn much more from Mark in the next two chapters about foods you can buy and prepare at home. But while you're at the restaurant Mark has a few great tips for making your experience a healthier one.

Since 3 percent of his customers have food allergies and an assortment of health concerns, Mark has been paying more attention to their needs. This trend seems to be nationwide, and more and more restaurants around the country are catering to the special requests of their clientele.

Can you ask the chef? While we don't recommend walking into the kitchen to ask him or her yourself, you can ask detailed questions of your service staff. If you're ordering beef, ask for a lean cut. When having fish, ask that it be simply prepared, without a lot of butter and sauce. Remember: get sauce served on the side so you can dip—a little. If the fish or chicken comes with a glaze, ask your waiter to keep it light and served on the side. If you have issues with salt, ask that the chef use a replacement, like herbs or an aromatic.

Don't be tentative. You're the customer, with every right to ask. Restaurants want return business, so if they can accommodate you, they will.

The Anatomy of a Salad

The basic salad you'll find in many fast-food and family restaurants is almost useless. All too often, food vendors use iceberg lettuce as the main ingredient, with a slice of tomato, a suggestion of cucumber, and a single strand of carrot. You can do better, especially when you ask your server to conjure up a few healthier and ultimately tastier ingredients in the kitchen.

If you're the shy type who doesn't want to bother your server, think again. Would you say, "I don't want to bother my doctor" if you didn't feel well because you ate too many bad salads? Look at it this way. If you're going to spend anywhere from $4.95 to $12.99 because you think it's supposed to be good for you, then at least make your money count for something healthy! Hint: if you're ever going to supersize anything, supersize your salad but not the dressing! Here's some sample dialogue to show you how easy it can be:

You: Hi, can I ask you a favor?

Server: Sure, what is it?

You: Well, the salad in the menu, see here in the picture.

Server: Uh huh.

You: Yeah, well there's a chunk of lettuce and a tomato slice and I don't know what this other thing is supposed to be.

Server: That's an onion ring. It must be there by mistake.

You: Oh my, could you hold the onion ring, please?

Server: Sure.

You: Thanks. Now, as far as my salad goes, do you think you could arrange for me to have a few vegetables in the bowl you bring me?

Server: What do you mean?

You: Well, you know what would be nice?

Server: What's that?

You: A couple more slices of tomato, a piece of cucumber, pepper, onion, and if you have some dark, leafy greens, like spinach, that would be terrific. You could hold the iceberg and just fill up my salad plate with spinach and vegetables. And some nuts if you have them, too, please.

Server: What kind of nuts?

You: Oh, some almonds or walnuts would be nice.

Server: I'll see what I can do.

You: And can I have the dressing on the side, please?

Server: On the side of what?

You: My plate. On the side of my plate here at the table.

Server: When I bring your food.

You: That's right.

Server: Sure.

The Wright Choice

You: Thanks so much. You know, this is really a much healthier salad you'll be serving. Doesn't that make you feel good?
Server: About what?
You: About playing a part in better health.
Server: I'm a waiter, not a doctor.
You: I know, I never meant to imply that you were. Nevermind.
Server: I'll get your salad now.
You: Thank you so much.
Server: Whatever.

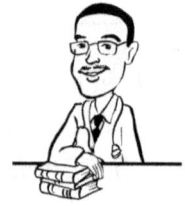

THE WRIGHT ADVICE
Many restaurants offer breadbaskets with butter.
Ask for a whole-grain option if you don't see one.
Ask for a butter substitute.
If it's sugar you need for coffee or tea, request a substitute.

The Cheaper the Menu, the Higher Your Cost in Health Care

Trying to save money? That's a good idea. But if a Quarter Pounder at McDonald's costs $1.49 and a bottle of Pepto-Bismol costs $3.99, then the total cost of your dinner is more than five dollars. Maybe some of these fast food restaurants could add an antacid drink to their menu so the cost would come down. On the other hand, maybe they could simply eliminate all those foods that cause us all this trouble in the first place.

I can dream, can't I? But even when you're trying to feed your family on a limited budget, you may want to reconsider where you eat. The money you think you might be saving at a fast-food joint may be only temporary when you consider the effects on your stomach and your skin and your heart. Teenagers already spend a small fortune on acne creams and blemish protectors. If they cut down on all the fatty, starchy foods they ate, they might save a nice little chuck of change on all those products.

On the other hand, if you're lucky enough to eat in a five-star establishment, you may not consider yourself so lucky once you calculate the amount of calories and fats you've ingested. But don't despair. Any restaurant worth its salt—or salt substitute—will have healthy options. Just like we recommended asking your server for healthy salad options in your average family restaurant, you can also ask your server in an upscale restaurant for the same choices.

Doggy Bag Nation

Drive by any family restaurant and you'll see folks in the parking lot walking to the car with a doggy bag. Why? Because in all probability, they have been served more food than they can or should eat at one sitting. We already know it's unhealthy for you or your children to overeat, so why not pack up the food you like and bring it home, put it in the frig, and save it for the next day?

It's a triple play. You'll have less food to prepare tomorrow. You'll get to enjoy, once again, the food you chose. And you'll save money!

Economizing at Home and On the Go

Doggie bags are just one idea for saving money when you're eating out. At home, there are countless ways to hold on to your hard-earned cash and still feed your family a delicious menu of excellent food. Surely you discovered quite a few items in your pantry that you probably never needed in the first place. Many of them may have already passed their expiration date. It's amazing how many things we buy that we never end up using. With some thoughtful planning you can minimize that and save yourself quite a bit of money. If you haven't already restocked your pantry with plenty of good, healthy foods, now is your chance to see how smart a shopper you can be.

In the next chapter, you'll discover how to plan many different types of meals, both to serve at home and to take with you for lunches, snacks, and family picnics. You'll have plenty of chances to use your new pantry items and to expand them, as well.

The best way to save money is by planning ahead and organizing what you will need to execute the menus you select. This not only eliminates waste, which saves money; it reduces all that decision making, saving you valuable time.

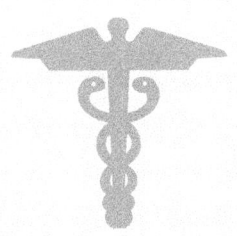

The Wright Reminders

No white bread.

No white sugar!

No processed lunchmeats!

Plan your pantry.

Shop smart and save money.

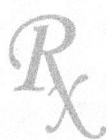

CHAPTER 13

Healthy Meals Made Easy: 50 Recipes to Feed Your Family

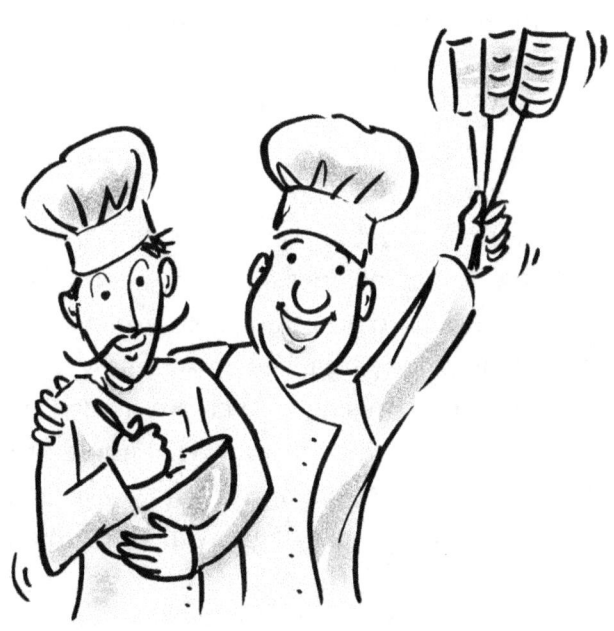

Healthy Home Cookin' on a Budget

As a doctor, it's my job to know as much as possible about food, nutrition, and the human body so I can make educated, constructive recommendations for my patients. Their health and my reputation are on the line each time I evaluate their conditions and prescribe a certain course of action intended to improve their health.

As a husband, father, and aspiring cook (my wife might dispute that), my motives might be somewhat different. I want to please my wife and kids with food they will enjoy, whether it's something I've made at home, bought in a store, or ordered in a restaurant. That desire to please is what can get all of us into trouble, because a mindset like that doesn't always lead to the kind of judgment that yields the best choices.

For example, my wife loves chocolate, and my kids adore hot dogs and ice cream. Now, I love my family and want to satisfy their whims, but should I really indulge them with such a triple threat to their health? If I do, is there a way of doing so that includes a healthy alternative? How about a smaller portion of slightly more expensive but better tasting chocolate? Perhaps I can serve my kids turkey hot dogs with no nitrites and ice cream made from tofu.

That can work with treats, but what about providing healthy meals at home that are easy to make and don't cost an arm and a leg? Let's begin with a healthy dose of realism. Most of you are looking for healthy alternatives for all those occasions when it's difficult to eat well. Plus, you want shopping to be easy and food preparation to be minimal, and you certainly don't want to sacrifice taste for good nutrition.

Houston chef Mark Holley, along with our consulting nutritionist, Anne Dubner, has created a healthy, delicious, and comprehensive meal plan designed to cover a family of four for three entire weeks. By following this menu, which is presented on pages 368 to 370, you will be forming positive and lasting food habits, and that's what it's all about. Of course, you may want to adapt it to fit you and your family. That means it may change according to the age of your kids, what food is available nearby, and your family schedule. Adapting the menu does not mean that you can simply add loads of salt, eat larger portions, or supplement everything with bacon.

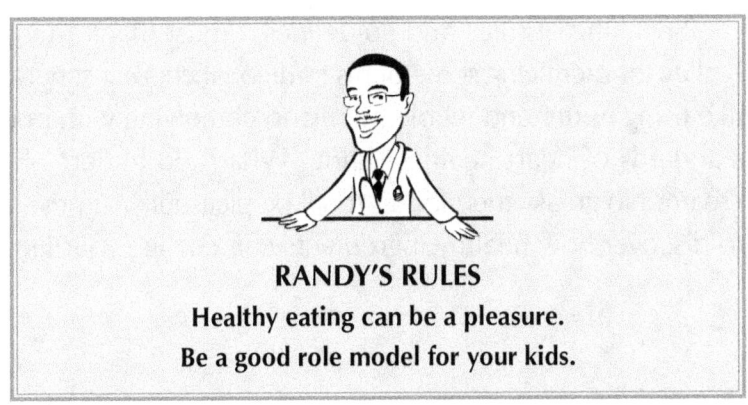

RANDY'S RULES
Healthy eating can be a pleasure.
Be a good role model for your kids.

Yummy Yummy and Heart Healthy, Too

Healthy food originates with good ingredients. I'm sure you'll be surprised to discover all the healthy options these recipes provide. It shouldn't be that difficult for you, as the adult in your family, to start changing the way you eat!

American Heart Association Recommendations

The American Heart Association recommends that everyone follow some basic rules, which will help you become intelligent and happy eaters. All of the recipes in this chapter follow these guidelines. But what do they mean? For example, how do the designated amounts translate into what we actually eat on a given day? With that in mind, we've asked Anne Dubner, our resident nutritionist and dietitian, to make sense of the food categories and their corresponding numbers. While each of us has different favorite foods, there can be no arguing the facts about what foods are best for us, as we have included here.

Speaking of rules and guidelines, I must thank Mark Holley for sacrificing some of his traditional chef's instincts, like using butter and whole milk, and complying with our standards of heart healthy eating. What? No butter? No cream? No greasy fried food? You'll be pleasantly surprised to discover how healthy ingredients can change your life.

AHA Food Groups and What They Mean for You

Fruits and vegetables: At least 4.5 cups a day.

What That Means:
The darker the color the better; they offer more health-enhancing antioxidants. One serving equals 1 cup raw or ½-cup cooked.

Fish (preferably oily fish): At least two 3.5-ounce servings a week.

What That Means:
Salmon, mackeral, sardines, and albacore tuna top the list. The omega-3 fatty acids in these selections help fight heart disease, stroke, and diabetes. One serving (the size of a deck of cards) equals 3.5 ounces, cooked. If you can find the "wild" variety with less chemicals, buy it.

Fiber-rich whole grains: At least three 1-ounce equivalent servings (uncooked) a day.

What That Means:
One serving equals a slice of bread, ⅓-cup of pasta or rice or other whole grain, a medium potato, ½-cup peas, corn, or beans. Whole grains provide B complex vitamins, which are important for keeping energy levels high. Fiber plays a vital role in keeping your digestive system running efficiently.

Sodium: Less than 1,500 milligrams a day.

What That Means:

One teaspoon of salt contains 2,300 milligrams of sodium, so use it sparingly, or, better yet, substitute other seasonings that do not contain salt at all. Experiment with different flavors, and you'll be surprised how you can create new and fresh varieties to your dishes. Many foods are naturally high in sodium, especially pickled and processed foods. When reading labels, look at the calorie count of the item per serving and then look at the sodium. It should not be more than two times the amount of calories. (If a soup contains 70 calories per serving, then the sodium should not total more than 140 milligrams.)

Sugar-sweetened beverages: No more than 450 calories (36 ounces) a week.

What That Means:

No more than 450 calories (36 ounces) a week! Sugar contributes nothing but trouble! It can lead to tooth decay, it aggravates diabetes, raises triglycerides, and it can lead to weight gain. Choose water as much as possible and squeeze some fresh lemon, lime, or other fruit into it to give it a "zing." Sugar enters the blood stream quickly, causing a boost of insulin to come along to counteract it. This sudden burst of "energy" can quickly result in as fast a drop in blood sugar as it has risen, causing fatigue.

Nuts, legumes, and seeds: At least 4 servings a week.

What That Means:

Nuts and seeds provide some protein and omega-3 fatty acids that are heart healthy. One serving of nuts or seeds is only about one tablespoon. Be careful of portion sizes if you are watching your weight, since only a small amount can add up quickly to many calories. For example, four walnut or pecan halves equal 45 calories. Legumes (like beans), on the other hand, are fat free, and four ½-cup servings a week will do you a world of good.

Processed meats: No more than 2 servings a week.

What That Means:

Read labels! Many processed meats have lots of salt and sugar added, not to mention other unknown substances. Some commercial brands do not contain artificial additives, but be prepared to pay a higher price. Why not make a chicken, turkey, or lean roast at home, where you can control what comes with it? 1 serving equals 3 ounces.

Saturated fat: Less than 7 percent of total energy intake.

What That Means:

Saturated fats are found in animal and some vegetable products (meats, butter, and hydrogenated vegetable oils). Limit portions to two teaspoons (about ten grams) at a time, and not more than three times per week. For example, a six-ounce hamburger (lean ground beef) without a bun contains eight grams of saturated fat.

FYI: Cholesterol is found only in animal products (beef, poultry, lamb, pork, etc.). While some foods may be labeled "No Cholesterol," many contain lots of saturated fats; for example, palm oil or coconut oil, which are high in fat but cholesterol free. I always say, "If it sounds like you can sit underneath it, then don't eat it!"

The Miracle of Planning Meals

Because many of us live such hectic lives, we have to be super organized. We may have our work clothes laid out the night before, our kid's laundry done, their after school classes set up, and our phones programmed with To Do lists to follow up on during the course of our working day. But what happens once we get home after a long day of work, errands, and soccer games? You walk in the door, put your briefcase down, and suddenly realize you have no idea what's in your refrigerator. Your kids are famished and asking what's for dinner. Honestly, you have no idea. It's a school night. You're not going out. Pizza sounds good, right? Maybe your spouse can pick up some burgers and fries on the way home.

Woops. Sounds like your options are going downhill fast. If only you'd planned ahead, even a little bit. You can. It's not a big deal. Some of you learned the virtues of being prepared back in the Boy Scouts. As parents, we're shockingly reminded about being prepared the first time we're away from home with a new baby and don't have a diaper handy. So why can't we learn to plan ahead for feeding our family? Wouldn't it be great to come home after a long, crazy day and walk into your kitchen with a plan? One or two hours on a Sunday evening preparing for the week ahead will pay huge dividends by midweek. That, along with smart shopping and planning your pantry, will enable you to make the most of these menus. Make meal planning your personal gift.

Mix and Match Leftovers

The meals presented here really add up to more than a month of menu choices when you consider simple modifications to basic recipes, leftover combinations, and your own personal flair.

When it comes to leftovers, some of us can draw on our childhood, and how our mothers recycled foods into new recipes or simply changed the outer appearance to fool us into thinking we were eating some new mysterious concoction. In my house, what mattered most was how it tasted. In your house, I hope you will combine taste with good health.

The extent of your culinary creativity is up to you. Cooking can be much more than mere drudgery and the fulfillment of a responsibility. It can be challenging and fun! So don't be shy about involving your spouse and your kids, even the little ones. If your kids are older, you'll be doing them a great favor by teaching them how to take care of themselves around the kitchen. One day, they'll be living on their own and the lessons they learn today will last a lifetime. Plus, a family that makes food together appreciates eating it a whole lot more.

Servings, Tips, and Keys

Each recipe indicates how many people it's intended to serve. These days, with late nights at work, after school activities, and community obligations, many families don't get a chance to eat together as often as they might like. With that in mind, we've developed recipes that feed a variety of family situations. You can easily adjust the amounts to fit your specific needs.

We are also providing some tips on multiple uses for some foods, ways to involve your children in preparation, and some novel ideas to keep your family engaged in healthy eating.

We're following up on the information we've presented in previous chapters about nutritional values, including calories, fat, carbohydrates, fiber, protein, sodium, and sugar. We're including a key code with each recipe, with numerical values for each of these categories so you can keep track of what you're eating.

Our intention with all of these recipes has been to keep the flavors high and the bad math low, meaning we want everything to be rich and tasty but it's just as important to keep calorie, fat, salt, and sugar counts to a minimum. It's like playing a game of nutritional limbo. How low can you go?

How the Key Code Works

Each recipe will include nutritional information in a thin box, which will look like this:

> **Nutrients Per Serving**
> **C** = 00 • **F** = 0g • **SF** = 0g • **CHO** = 0mg • **CAR** = 0g • **FI** = 0g
> **P** = 00g • **SO** = 00mg • **S** = 0g

C = Calories	**F** = Fat (total)	**SF** = Saturated Fats
CHO = Cholesterol	**CAR** = Carbohydrates	**FI** = Fiber
P = Protein	**SO** = Sodium	**S** = Sugar

> **Additional information is available at our website:**
> **www.TheWrightChoiceRx.com**

The Semantics of Recipes

"As needed" means only when really needed. For example, if you need to add a bit of honey, add a bit, not half a bottle. Common sense can go a long way.

"To taste" means use your better judgment when adding simple seasoning. For example, many recipes include salt and pepper. In our nutritional analysis, we have not included any calculations for salt content. But keep in mind there are 2,300 milligrams of sodium in one teaspoon of salt.

"Drizzle" means drip, as in a little bit!

Replacing Old Favorites with New (Healthy) Options

You'll see that we've replaced traditional staples with healthier alternatives. For example, instead of full-fat butter, we're using butter substitutes, which are not the same as margarine. Why? Because margarine has additives, and the many butter substitutes on the market today are much healthier. As for cooking in butter—forget it! As much as this pained our chefs, we recommend non-fat cooking spray, which can be found as safflower, canola, or olive oil, all suitable for cooking.

As the recipes unfold, you'll discover many other healthy alternatives.

Dr. Wright's Recipes
for
Busy Families On the Go

50 Quick 'n' Easy Recipes

from

Chef Mark Holley
(PESCE)

with

Guest Recipes

from

David Cordua
(Americas)

Houston's Up-and-Coming Chef of 2010

A Special Thanks

It's an honor to have chefs Mark Holley and David Cordua sharing their recipes with us. I am also thankful for enjoying their friendship outside of their respective kitchens.

Mark, the executive chef of PESCE, one of Houston's award-winning restaurants, worked tirelessly to ensure that we are providing delicious and healthy meals for all of you. That wasn't always easy, however, because Mark, like most chefs, was trained in the world of food chemistry and gourmet flavors, which means taste comes first, and nutritional values are often an afterthought. As a result, we had some battles over using butter and milk and various oils, etc. Sometimes, Anne Dubner and I even had to join forces to convince Mark that we could still feed people well without raising their cholesterol levels to sky-high proportions. This process created quite a learning curve for all of us. I'd also like to thank Mark's sous chefs, Patrick Blackman and William Thompson, for their dedication to this project and their perpetual good cheer.

David, whose father, Michael Cordua, has been inducted into *Food & Wine* magazine's Hall of Fame, has developed quite a reputation of his own through his family's restaurants in Houston. He was named the 2010 Up-and-Coming Chef of the Year in Houston by *My Table* magazine. We are grateful for the recipes David has contributed and appreciate his willingness to adapt certain ingredients to fit our nutritional standards.

These recipes met my standards and those of professional nutritionist and dietitian Anne Dubner, a former national spokesperson for the American Dietetic Association and a mother of two, who practices in the Houston area. With more than 30 years of experience teaching parents and children about wholesome food choices, Anne offers practical advice on how to provide well-rounded meals and snacks. She has supervised every recipe in this chapter to ensure that its nutritional content meets the standards of the American Heart Association.

With an eye to the future and improving the eating habits of our kids, I have asked Anne to answer some questions regarding our children's health and their relationships to food. I'm quite sure her answers will be as helpful for you as they have been for me. Look for those discussions throughout this chapter. And now—THE FOOD!

Breakfast!

From Breakfast on the Run to Lazy Brunches

During the course of a workweek, our eating habits vary. Most families are in a rush on school days, and things slow down sometimes at dinner and hopefully more often on the weekends. Chef Holley recognizes all of that and wants to satisfy the average family's need to accommodate all of these demands and preferences. You'll find many useful and entertaining ideas to turn your daily diet into a healthy and positive experience.

You'll also notice that we're not trying to turn anyone into an overnight health nut who will run a marathon by the time he finishes reading this book. That means keeping in mind our busy schedules and the desire to enjoy the foods we like, we've included a range of recipes that simultaneously educate and indulge. Use your best judgment in determining how you blend these foods into your weekly eating plans.

Five Breakfasts in 10 Minutes or Less

All of these recipes can be made quickly and easily, and if your children are old enough, why not make them responsible for making breakfast at least once a week? When children take ownership of their eating, they tend to grow up with a better appreciation for food, both its meaning and its day-to-day sustenance.

Starting the Day with Randy and Anne

Randy: *With school starting so early in the morning, what can we offer our kids when they may not be hungry so that they start the day eating something healthy?*

Anne: My girls are in ninth and fifth grade so I know that issue. We love to make mini muffins (corn, blueberry, carrot, etc) in advance. With a small cup of a yogurt smoothie (see recipe on page 289), it's a light, healthy, and delicious way to start the day. Not to mention conveniently quick because I don't know about you but we always seem to be in a rush in the morning.

Randy: *Yeah, that's part of the reason we decided to focus this book on busy families.*

Anne: Right! We've got great recipes here that should satisfy everyone's schedule and palette.

Randy: *They should be going off to school happy and well fed.*

Anne: Make sure that you send your children to school with some snacks, too, such as crackers, cheese, yogurt, fruit, or cold cereal, in case they get hungry later in the day.

Randy: *We cover those, too, coming up in this chapter.*

Cherry Oatmeal
(Serves 4)

2 cups water
pinch of salt
1 cup quick oats
½ teaspoon ground cinnamon

½ cup sliced bananas
2 tablespoons dried cherries
honey or agave syrup

What to Do

1. Place water in a 2-quart pot and add a pinch of salt. Bring to a boil, and add oats and cinnamon. Lower heat, cover pot (oatmeal likes steam), and let simmer for 5 to 8 minutes, stirring occasionally.

2. Remove from heat and fold in bananas, cherries, and a drizzle of honey or agave syrup. Can be served hot or cold.

TIP: If you use (organic) skimmed milk (which is handy for those kids who don't like to drink milk), pay close attention that it doesn't scald as it's heating up. Skim milk is also a healthy way to cool off the oatmeal quickly for serving.

Enjoy with the morning paper or while quizzing your son for his chemistry test.

Nutrients Per Serving
C = 112 • **F** = 2g • **SF** = 0g • **CHO** = 0mg • **CAR** = 22g • **FI** = 3g
P = 3g • **SO** = 74mg • **S** = 7g

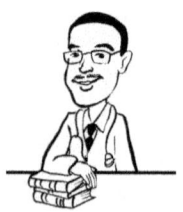

THE WRIGHT ADVICE
Oatmeal is a cholesterol friendly food and highly recommended.
Limit the agave syrup or honey to one teaspoon.
Modify your sweet tooth, one breakfast at a time.

Crepe Ambrosia with Sauce Ala Orange
aka
French Pancake with Orange Sauce
(Serves 4)

Crepe

8 ounces egg substitute
1 egg yolk
10 ounces water
8 ounces skimmed milk
4 tablespoons butter substitute, melted

1½ oz granulated sugar
½ teaspoon salt
8 ounces all-purpose flour, sifted
vegetable spray

What to Do

1. In a small bowl, whisk together egg substitute, egg yolk, water, and milk. Stir in melted butter substitute (best to melt in microwave oven).

2. Add sugar, salt, and flour, and whisk together. Heat a nonstick frying pan and coat lightly with vegetable spray. Pour 2½ ounces (a single crepe portion) of batter into pan and swirl to coat the bottom evenly. Cook crepe until it sets and turns light brown (approximately 60 seconds).

Filling

½ cup low-fat cream cheese (room temperature)
¼ cup plain, non-fat yogurt
½ teaspoon lemon juice, freshly squeezed
½ teaspoon honey or agave syrup

2 tablespoons pecans, chopped
2 tablespoons sundried cherries
2 tablespoons apples, diced small
2 tablespoons coconut flakes, unsweetened

What to Do

1. Combine cream cheese (room temperature), yogurt, lemon juice, honey or agave syrup, and mix well. Fold in remaining ingredients and mix well.

TIP: The key to easy mixing is using cream cheese at room temperature.

Nutrients Per Serving
C = 564 • **F** = 23g • **SF** = 10g • **CHO** = 85mg • **CAR** = 73g • **FI** = 9g
P = 22g • **SO** = 722mg • **S** = 23g

Sauce Ala Orange
(Serves 4)

3 tablespoons sugar
1 teaspoon cornstarch
¾ cup orange juice

1 tablespoon brandy
2 tablespoons chopped orange sections (optional)
mint sprigs

What to Do

1. In a small bowl, combine sugar and cornstarch and set aside. In a small sauté pan, over medium heat, add orange juice and brandy and bring to a simmer. Stir in the sugar and cornstarch mixture you just made and cook it until the sauce has thickened, stirring occasionally. Remove from heat and stir in orange sections if you prefer.

Note: When cooking brandy, nearly all of the alcohol actually burns away. If you have young children, you may choose to omit the brandy. Then again, if you have a lot of *young* children, you may choose to add more. (Joke!)

2. Place crepe rolls onto a plate in a crisscross pattern. Pour sauce over crepes and garnish with mint.

Nutrients Per Serving
C = 70 • **F** = 0g • **SF** = 0g • **CHO** = 0mg • **CAR** = 15g • **FI** = 0g
P = 0g • **SO**= 1mg • **S** = 14g

"Crepe"
A Guide to Proper Pronunciation

First of all, it's not *crap*, as in you know what. That would be too silly and much too easy a target for France busters. And it's not *crape*, as in what Batman wears, only with an R. Finally, it's not *creep*, as in people who hang around 7-11 parking lots.

It's crepe—rhymes with rep, as in the reputation we Americans have for butchering the French language.

Speaking of butchering things French: if, by the end of making this recipe your crepe looks more like an omelet, then it's an omelet. But you can play it safe and call it by its French name—Omelet!

ChefSpeak

You've probably noticed that we don't use any brand names in our recipes. That's intentional. While some brands are nationally known, many are regional or local and we don't want to create any confusion or unnecessary competition. It's up to you to investigate what's available in your area, and once you've educated yourself about what your community offers, you can make the best choices of what to purchase.

Be open-minded. The barrage of television advertising and circulars in your local paper is meant to convince you, without you even knowing it, that you just can't live without certain products. Truth is, you can live much better without many of them.

Are Your Nuts Too Fatty?

All this talk about fats in our foods can be misleading. It all depends on the source of the fat in question. As you discovered in Chapter 8, for example, some nuts are full of heart healthy fats. Salmon and other fish may sound like they're high in fat when we first hear the numbers, but upon closer inspection we discover that the omega-rich fats found in fish are a positive thing to be eating. It's a good idea to check the overall percentage of fats in whatever foods you are eating. That will determine the appropriate dosage and frequency for eating.

The Wright Choice

Morning Alert! Two on the Go—Preparation Needed!

I know what it's like to run out of time in the morning and race out of the house without a thing in my stomach. Halfway to work I'm not paying attention to the road because I'm so hungry. If I pull over to buy something, I'll be late. Plus, I'll probably end up buying some pretty unhealthy food, woolf it down, and end up with a bad stomachache by the time I get to work.

Following are two wonderful alternatives to make at home, with about two hours of free time and some help from your family.

Power Bar
(Serves 8)

cooking spray
1 cup chopped pecans
½ cup sliced almonds
½ cup shredded coconut
2 cups oatmeal
3 cups puffed rice

½ cup sundried cherries
½ teaspoon ground cinnamon
½ cup honey
½ cup light corn syrup
½ teaspoon salt
½ teaspoon vanilla extract

What to Do

1. Preheat oven to 350°F. and lightly coat baking pan with cooking spray. In a small bowl, combine pecans, almonds, and coconut. Spread onto baking pan and cook for 5 to 7 minutes, stirring occasionally. Let it cook until coconut is light brown. Remove from pan and place in a small bowl. Add oats, puffed rice, sundried cherries, and cinnamon. Mix well. Set aside.

2. Combine honey, corn syrup, salt, and vanilla in a saucepan over medium heat. Simmer for 5 minutes, stirring occasionally.

3. Stir syrup mixture over oatmeal mixture and mix well.

4. Lightly coat a 1½-quart glass baking pan with cooking spray and pour in mixture. Press down firmly with one hand until it flattens in the pan. Let it sit for 15 to 20 minutes to cool. Turn the pan upside down and gently tap the top until the mixture falls onto a cutting board. Cut into 8 pieces or as desired, depending on the ages of your kids.

TIP: You'll notice that these finished power bars are drier and not so abundantly sweet like the ones you buy commercially. That's because they don't have the syrupy, sugar-laced binders like the others, which make them all so gooey and tight.

Nutrients Per Serving
C = 445 • F = 19g • SF = 4g • CHO = 0mg • CAR = 65g • FI = 6g
P = 8g • SO = 175mg • S = 32g

What About Cooking Spray?

There are many different types available. We recommend non-fat versions, such as safflower, sunflower, canola, or olive oil. Check the packaging information for oils that are suitable for high heat cooking. If you purchase organic products, those are preferable. They're a bit more expensive in most cases, but these are products that last a long time and the extra cost is well worth it.

Granola

(Serves 4)

(This recipe will yield approximately two sandwich bags of granola.)

1 2/3 cup uncooked oats
½ cup unsweetened coconut flakes
¼ cup sliced almonds
¼ cup chopped pecans
¼ teaspoon salt
¼ teaspoon ground cinnamon

1 tablespoon vegetable oil
2 tablespoons honey
¼ cup dried cherries
¼ cup raisins
¼ cup chopped dried apricots

What to Do

1. Preheat oven to 250°F. In a large bowl, combine oats, coconut, almonds, pecans, salt, and cinnamon.

2. In a separate bowl, combine oil and honey. Combine both mixtures and spread onto a baking pan. Bake for 1½ hours, stirring every 15 minutes with a spatula. Add cherries, raisins, and apricots and mix well.

Nutrients Per Serving

C = 345 • **F** = 12g • **SF** = 2g • **CHO** = 0mg • **CAR** = 54g • **FI** = 7g
P = 8g • **SO** = 153mg • **S** = 26g

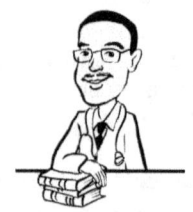

THE WRIGHT ADVICE

Power bars and granola are not only great
for an emergency portable breakfast,
they work in lunchboxes, picnic boxes,
backpacks, glove compartments, etc.

Keep them on hand as a snack, hiking partner, or to keep siblings
happy in the backseat on those long drives to your in-laws.

Your Very Own Smoothie Bar

We discussed shakes and healthy drinks in Chapter 7 and how they can provide good sources of protein, vitamins, and necessary minerals. Those elements are provided by powders and can be mixed with water, juices, or milk. Why not take that a step further and create flavorful, delicious, and healthy smoothies for your whole family? You can serve them anytime. You can even pour them into a thermos and include them in your lunchbox. Welcome to your very own smoothie bar.

Smoothie
(Serves 1)

4 ounces bananas	4 ounces strawberries
1 tablespoon honey	1 cup non-fat skim milk
½ cup plain non-fat yogurt	2 tablespoons low-fat granola

What to Do

1. Combine all ingredients in a blender and process until smooth. Vary fruits according to taste.

TIP: You can substitute water for milk or mix with a small amount of juice. Add protein powder if you prefer. A tablespoon won't make it too thick. Portion size can be adjusted to suit the ages of your children.

Nutrients Per Serving
C = 398 • **F** = 2g • **SF** = 1g • **CHO** = 7mg • **CAR** = 85g • **FI** = 6g
P = 18g • **SO** = 238mg • **S** = 67g

BEST BLENDERS

You could spend hundreds of dollars for a machine that claims it can change your life. Or you can buy a decent blender that makes an excellent protein smoothie and have money to spare for more genuine pleasures.

Buckwheat Blueberry Pancakes
(Serves 4)

½ cup buckwheat flour
½ cup all-purpose flour
1 tablespoon brown sugar
2 tablespoons baking powder
½ teaspoon salt
cooking spray

¾ cup soy milk
2 tablespoons vegetable oil
2 tablespoons egg white
1 cup blueberries
agave syrup

What to Do

1. In a small bowl, combine buckwheat flour, all-purpose flour, brown sugar, baking powder, and salt. Mix well. Hum your favorite tune.

2. In a separate bowl, whisk together soy milk, oil, and egg white.

3. Pour wet mixture into dry mixture only until blended.

4. Lightly coat a griddle (preferred) or nonstick frying pan with cooking spray and heat until hot. Drop two tablespoons of batter onto hot griddle for each pancake. Drop blueberries on top of each pancake. Turn pancakes when bubbly and cook 2 to 3 minutes. Drizzle with agave syrup and serve immediately.

Warning

These pancakes, because of the buckwheat flour, will not look like the golden brown pancakes you may be used to eating at IHOP. That's because buckwheat not only tastes good, it's good for you.

Nutrients Per Serving
C = 218 • **F** = 8g • **SF** = 1g • **CHO** = 0mg • **CAR** = 32g • **FI** = 3g
P = 00g • **SO** = 658mg • **S** = 3g

The 12-Hour Window of Opportunity

If you make pancake batter beforehand and refrigerate it, make sure you observe the 12-hour window rule: Do not store pancake batter more than 12 hours before using it to make pancakes. Pretty straightforward, wouldn't you say? But if you want an alternative, prepare the wet and dry ingredients separately, store them like that, and combine them only when you are ready to cook the pancakes.

Brunch!

Leisurely (Lazy) Brunch Recipes

These recipes are great for those slow, weekend days when no one in the family is rushing off to school or work. If you find that you're rushing around the house anyway, mindlessly programmed by our hyped-up society to keep busy at all times, here's your chance to slow down and give your body and soul a chance to recharge. Taking your time in the kitchen to prepare food slowly, with love and attention, is an excellent tonic for combating our frantic lifestyles. Do yourself a favor and learn to enjoy this time. You and your family will all enjoy the benefits.

Mediterranean Latkes
(Serves 4)

- 1 pound finely grated raw potatoes
- 1 tablespoon all purpose flour
- 2 tablespoons egg white
- 2 tablespoons roasted garlic (optional)
- 2 tablespoons olive oil
- cooking spray
- ¾ cup egg substitute
- 2 tablespoons feta cheese, crumbled
- 2 tablespoons roasted peppers, chopped
- 2 tablespoons basil, chopped
- salt/pepper to taste

What to Do

1. Preheat oven to 350°F. Grate potatoes and rinse well with cold water. Place them onto a cloth towel and squeeze well until all the moisture is removed. Place in a small bowl. Fold in flour, egg white, and roasted garlic (recipe on next page) and mix well.

2. In a large, nonstick frying pan, add 2 tablespoons of oil over high heat. Pour in entire mixture to fill the frying pan as one large pancake. Flatten with spatula. Cook 2 to 3 minutes on each side or until golden brown. Place pan in oven for 5 to 7 minutes. Remove from pan and drain on a paper towel.

3. In a small, nonstick sauté pan over medium heat, lightly coat with cooking spray and scramble egg substitute until light and frothy.

To serve, place scrambled eggs over the giant latke. Sprinkle with feta cheese, roasted peppers, and chopped basil. Add salt and pepper.

Nutrients Per Serving
$C = 204 \cdot F = 0g \cdot SF = 2g \cdot CHO = 4mg \cdot CAR = 0g \cdot FI = 2g$
$P = 9g \cdot SO = 191mg \cdot S = 3g$

Roasted Garlic

Garlic is known for its olfactory powers (as in "Wo! Who here ate garlic?"), but did you know that garlic plays an important role in reducing blood pressure, cholesterol, and hypertension? With that in mind, here are three ways to use roasted garlic as a wonderful part of your cooking experience.

> *"You can never have enough garlic.*
> *With enough garlic, you can eat* The New York Times.*"*
> Morley Safer

Preheat your oven to 350°F and prepare a baking dish. Gather a few heads of garlic, depending on how much you want to prepare. All three garlic concoctions we're presenting here can be nicely kept in the refrigerator, so we advise you to make more than you need for any one recipe. There will be plenty of occasions to use it later.

Purple striped garlic is well known for its sweetness, which is great for baking, but any type of garlic will do. Start by removing about half an inch from the heads of the garlic, leaving each clove exposed so that later on it will be easy to squeeze out the mushy insides. Keep the skins right where they are.

Place the garlic cloves in the dish. If you are a true garlic lover, you'll throw in the tops that you just cut off but watch out—they burn easily. Check them while cooking.

Drizzle the garlic with olive oil, letting it drip in between the cloves. Cover your dish with aluminum foil so the edges are tight. Roast for 30 to 45 minutes, checking after 20 minutes to be sure no little pieces are burning. Make sure you wrap the foil tightly afterward.

The garlic is done when it turns light brown and becomes mushy soft. To be sure, poke it with a fork. Remove each clove with a small knife or squeeze until the cloves pop out. Let the party begin!

What About That Leftover Garlic Oil?

Good question. Take your baking dish and pour any remaining olive oil through a strainer into a small bowl. Press what's left of the garlic with a spoon to squeeze any extra oil out. The garlic oil will keep in the refrigerator for about a week. When you want to enjoy it, let it come to room temperature before using.

> "A nickel will get you on the subway, but garlic will get you a seat."
> Old New York proverb

Roasted Garlic Butter

Take 8 tablespoons of butter substitute and let it soften in a bowl for 20 minutes. The amount of butter substitute you need depends on how much garlic you roasted and how much of it you want to mix into a paste. Then there's the question of how strong you prefer your concoction.

In any case, take a fork and make a paste of the butter substitute and garlic. If it seems too loose, don't worry; it will become firm once it gets cold.

Take a piece of waxed paper or parchment paper. Place your mixture on top and roll it into a log. Twist the ends up tightly to keep it sealed and put in the refrigerator for a few hours. It should turn into regular-looking butter, but it will sure smell a lot more interesting! You can use it for a variety of purposes. If you keep it well sealed, it will last for a few weeks. Enjoy!

> "Stop and smell the garlic! That's all you have to do."
> William Shatner

Healthy Meals Made Easy: 50 Recipes to Feed Your Family

Smoked Salmon Omelet
(Serves 4)

cooking spray
1/3 cup raw asparagus, chopped
2 tablespoons red onion, diced small
4 ounces smoked salmon, chopped
2 teaspoons dry dill weed, chopped
1 cup egg substitute

What to Do

1. Using a nonstick omelet pan, spray well with olive oil cooking spray. Over medium high heat, sauté asparagus and red onions for 2 minutes. Remove from heat. Add smoked salmon and dill. Mix well and place onto a plate.

2. Using the same pan, over medium heat, pour in egg mixture. With a rubber spatula, push eggs gently until firm. Add salmon mixture on top of eggs and fold eggs over to form an omelet. Play French national anthem on nose flute.

Once that is complete and omelet has set, place it on a plate. Eat and enjoy.

Nutrients Per Serving
C = 68 • F = 1g • SF = 10 • CHO = 7mg • CAR = 2g • FI = 0g
P = 12g • SO = 693mg • S = 1g

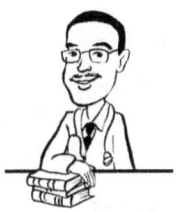

THE WRIGHT ADVICE

While you're waiting for your kids to make it from the TV to the table, cover the omelets to keep them warm. You can garnish the omelet with cherry tomatoes, and if they still haven't shown up, an alarm clock might be advisable.
If you decide to add a cream cheese twist, use tofu cream cheese. Try not telling anyone and see if she even notices.

Turkey Pita with Tomato Relish
(Serves 4)

cooking spray
2 tablespoons red onions, chopped
4 ounces ground turkey sausage
1 cup egg substitute
4 whole-wheat pita breads
2 ounces lite mozzarella cheese, grated
tomato relish (see below)

What to Do

1. Pre-heat oven to 325°F. Lightly coat a non stick frying pan with cooking spray and place over medium-high heat. Add onions and turkey sausage, and cook for 4 minutes or until sausage is completely cooked.

2. Remove from pan and set aside.

3. Spray skillet again with cooking spray and place over medium heat. Beat eggs in a small bowl. Scramble eggs in pan. Warm pitas in oven for 5 minutes, remove, and divide scrambled eggs among the pitas. Stuff each with sausage mixture, cheese, and tomato relish (see below).

Nutrients Per Serving
$C = 299$ • $F = 7g$ • $SF = 5g$ • $CHO = 28mg$ • $CAR = 40g$ • $FI = 5g$
$P = 22g$ • $SO = 800mg$ • $S = 3g$

Tomato Relish

½ cup yellow cherry tomatoes, sliced
2 tablespoons red onions, chopped
½ lime, freshly squeezed
½ cup red cherry tomatoes
2 teaspoons cilantro, chopped
salt/pepper to taste

What to Do

Play your favorite music. Combine all ingredients in a bowl and mix well.

Quesadilla Margherita
(Serves 2)

cooking spray
½ ounces Parmesan cheese, shredded
2 whole-wheat tortillas, 8-inch
3 ounces lite mozzarella cheese, shredded
1 teaspoon basil, julienne (chopped)
2.5 ounces Roma tomato, diced

What to Do

1. Lightly coat a nonstick frying pan with cooking spray and bring to medium heat.

2. Sprinkle the pan with half of the Parmesan cheese. Place the bottom tortilla in the pan and add mozzarella, basil, tomato, and second tortilla on top.

3. Lower the heat to allow cheese to melt and tortilla to lightly brown. Flip and lightly brown other tortilla.

4. Remove and slice into 4 pieces and garnish with remaining Parmesan cheese. Serve with your favorite organic salsa.

Note on Servings

In a restaurant, when you order this dish, you'd normally receive two quesadilla on your plate. That's a whole lot of fat, etc. But at home, where you're at the mercy of only your own decisions, you can choose to eat just one!

Nutrients Per Serving
C = 221 • **F** = 9g • **SF** = 6g • **CHO** = 30mg • **CAR** = 23g • **FI** = 2g
P = 17g • **SO** = 504mg • **S** = 2g

This recipe is courtesy of David Cordua from *Churascos* in Houston.

Some of its ingredients have been adapted for this book.

One Pot Breakfast
(Serves 4)

1½ cups skim milk	4 slices chopped turkey bacon, cooked
½ cup water	½ cup chopped asparagus, blanched
1½ cups grits	½ cup low-fat cheddar cheese
¼ cup frozen corn	salt/pepper to taste

What to Do

1. In a saucepan, add milk and water. Bring to a boil. Stir in grits, lower heat, and cover. Let simmer for 4 minutes.

2. Sprinkle in corn, turkey bacon, chopped asparagus, and shredded cheese. Cover and continue to cook on low heat for 7 to 10 minutes.

3. Remove from heat, let it sit for 5 minutes, and serve.

Nutrients Per Serving
C = 327 • **F** = 5g • **SF** = 2g • **CHO** = 17mg • **CAR** = 55g • **FI** = 2g
P = 15g • **SO** = 362mg • **S** = 6g

Blanched—What's That Mean?

Just as your child may blanch (turn pale) at the idea of eating asparagus, that's exactly what you'll be doing when you blanch a vegetable. It's simply the act of boiling them: to whiten, to remove skin, to rid them of strong flavors, or prepare them for freezing.

According to Chef Holley, after boiling your vegetables in lightly salted water for 2 to 3 minutes (or until barely done), place them in an ice water mixture. Remove them as soon as they are no longer warm. You can re-heat them however you'd like.

Salt Substitutes

While this recipe is not particularly high in sodium, others may be, and for those with high blood pressure, hypertension, or other issues, it's important to control your salt intake. Nowadays, you can find excellent salt substitutes in your local grocery store. Ask your doctor what he or she recommends or check with a dietitian at your children's school.

Frittata
(Serves 2)

3 cups water
½ cup chopped asparagus, blanched
olive oil cooking spray
1 tablespoon garlic, chopped
¼ cup scallions (bulbs and greens), chopped
½ cup raw whole mushrooms, sliced
2 tablespoons Parmesan cheese, grated
¾ cup egg substitute
2 tablespoons lite mozzarella, grated
salt/pepper to taste

What to Do

1. Preheat oven to 350°F. In a small saucepan, add 3 cups of water and bring to a boil. Add asparagus and cook for 2 minutes. Remove from heat and strain. Rinse with cold water to chill. Set aside.

2. In a medium nonstick sauté pan, coat well with olive oil cooking spray. Sauté garlic and scallions for 2 minutes. Add mushrooms and sauté for 4 more minutes. Add asparagus and mix well. Remove from heat and stir in Parmesan cheese.

3. In a nonstick frying pan over medium heat, add egg substitute. Cook, without stirring, for 3 minutes. Add mushroom and asparagus on top. Place pan in oven for 3 minutes. Remove from oven, sprinkle with mozzarella cheese, return to oven, and cook 3 more minutes. Slide frittata onto large plate and serve.

Nutrients Per Serving
C = 165 • **F** = 8g • **SF** = 3g • **CHO** = 9mg • **CAR** = 8g • **FI** = 1g
P = 16g • **SO** = 365mg • **S** = 7g

Do Your Children Suffer from "Vegetable Allergies?"

It's the asparagus, right? We thought that might pose a risk for families with young children or stubborn adults. Don't worry. You have options! Choose a different vegetable. Choose more than one. You can rarely go wrong with too many vegetables in a dish, especially when it comes to nutritional value. Go green if you can, as in broccoli, kale, or peppers. Let your kids get involved. This breakfast is a great way to involve them in the cooking process.

Nana's Leftovers

Save money. Save time. Save the environment. Honor your grandmother.

What historians refer to as the study of "ancient leftovers" began in a cave in the Himalayas in the year 33, when cave men and women traditionally cooked a single, large sloth, and, after its initial serving, continued eating it as leftovers until they literally grew sick of it and expired. This era also marks the origins of the word "sloth," which originally signified one who simply was too lazy to hunt anything else and continued eating the same animal, in this case a sloth, until his or her body rejected it.

What does this have to do with leftovers? Well, with all the time you save recycling those good dinners and lunches, you will have time to do this kind of research and dazzle your offspring with your newfound knowledge.

STOP!

EXERCISE BREAK!

I'm guessing that reading these delicious recipes has gotten you out of your chair and into the kitchen to raid your refrigerator—at least once.

That's all fine and good, but it means it's time to exercise for 30 minutes.

Eat less.

Exercise more.

Didn't I hear that someplace recently?

Lunch!

A Lunchbox for School and the Office

Your children go to school approximately 180 days a year, and that's a lot of lunches! It's at least the same for parents, and those midday meals are important, for our health and our pocketbooks. Hopefully, they aren't depleting either of them, but truth be told, I've heard from too many people—of all economic backgrounds—that they struggle with providing healthy, affordable lunches for themselves and their children.

Let's take care of that right now.

Five Lunchboxes for Kids of All Ages

With the national debate heating up on children's nutrition it's about time we pay better attention to what our children are eating—at home, on the road, and in school. The recipes in this section pay tribute to some good, old-fashioned traditions, as well as introducing a few new ideas—for the head and palette. We hope you will encourage your kids to try new foods and pay attention themselves to making healthier choices.

Lunchbox Science with Randy and Anne

Each August and September, as summer winds down and a new school year approaches, millions of families go searching for the perfect lunchbox for their children, as if finding their favorite characters with the coolest thermos inside will make life good. But wait. What about the food that goes inside those lunchboxes (or brown bags, for those of you more inclined to "old school" it)? Who's paying attention to what your kids are eating in school each day? You're a busy parent so we've got you covered with Anne Dubner, aka The Food Cop.

Randy: *How much should you pack in an average lunch?*

Anne: Parents often believe that children need to have many items in their lunch. I know several moms who send 10 items or more, in the hope that the child will eat "something." Please resist the urge to do this! Don't overwhelm your child with too many choices. Have two to three items, perhaps a sandwich (one of those here in the book), along with a piece of fruit and some pretzels or whole-grain crackers.

Randy: *Too much food in the middle of the day isn't healthy.*

Anne: Plus, it's simply wasteful.

Randy: *What about dessert?*

Anne: You're bad! Try to leave the sweet desserts at home, since your child will probably go for that first at school, leaving little room for the more healthy choices you provided.

Kids!

Peanut Butter Tea Sandwiches
(Serves 2)

Are you kidding me—tea sandwiches for my kids? Absolutely. They represent variety and reinforce portion control. My two little boys seem to prefer things that are their size, food included. I'm sure little girls do, too. And, I've seen kids of both genders in nursery schools, pretending to have tea parties. If I were you, I might even consider finding the chance to sit down and join them sometime.

peanut butter, low-fat (organic smooth) 1 banana
4 pieces whole-wheat bread 1 small apple or 1 strawberry
1 pear, cored and shredded

What to Do

1. Spread peanut butter on both slices of bread. Add whichever fruits you prefer, perhaps two in combination, depending on your children's (and your) taste. Cut into small, bite-sized pieces for easy eating. These sandwiches can work well for after-school snacks, too. Nutritional values vary a bit, depending on which fruits you use.

Nutrients Per Serving
C = 332 • **F** = 13g • **SF** = 2g • **CHO** = 0mg • **CAR** = 45g • **FI** = 7g
P = 13g • **SO** = 443mg • **S** = 13g

More Lunchbox Science with Randy and Anne

Randy: *How important is it to include fruits and vegetables in our children's diets?*

Anne: Fruits and veggies provide important nutrients for proper growth, so it is very important to include them as consistently as possible, even in lunchboxes.

Randy: *It can be tough to choose what's best for them.*

Anne: You can empower your child by having him choose which fruit or veggie he wants in his lunch. That will increase the chance of him eating it and not swapping it out for another child's cookie.

Randy: *What about dressings and dips to accompany the veggies?*

Anne: There are many yogurt dips available for fruits, and low-fat dips for veggies. A small amount of dip or dressing (and I stress the word "small") can increase the chances of your child actually eating the fruits and veggies you send to school.

Randy: *What about drinks? How do you feel about juice or sports drinks?*

Anne: Milk and water are the best choices. Fruit juices and sports drinks often have sugar added and don't offer the best nutrition. Even if a fruit drink is 100 percent juice, it's still better to eat the real thing—whole fruit—as dessert, for extra fiber.

Trail Mix Cracker
(Serves 2)

2 tablespoons low-fat cream cheese
1 teaspoon lemon juice
¼ teaspoon lemon zest
agave syrup, as needed

⅓ cup standard trail mix, chopped
2 tablespoons carrots, shredded
4 whole-wheat crackers

What to Do

1. In a small mixing bowl, add cream cheese (room temperature), lemon juice, and lemon zest and mix well. Wait. What's lemon zest? Simple. Take your lemon and a paring knife. Scrape off enough of the yellow skin to fill 1 teaspoon. That's lemon zest. Add trail mix and carrots and blend together. Spread 1 tablespoon of mixture on cracker, drizzle a drop of agave syrup, and serve.

Note: If you're not partial to lemons, use an equivalent amount of pineapple juice or soy milk.

Nutrients Per Serving
C = 175 • **F** = 10g • **SF** = 3g • **CHO** = 8mg • **CAR** = 17g • **FI** = 1g
P = 6g • **SO** = 143mg • **S** = 2g

MilkSpeak from Randy and Anne

Randy: *Should kids be drinking skim, 2%, or whole milk?*

Anne: If a child is overweight, skim or low-fat milk may be introduced after age two. If the child has no problem with weight, then whole milk is fine. Of course, portion control is crucial. Children need three 8-ounce cups of milk per day to provide adequate calcium. Studies have found that children who are given skim milk in their early years tend to have higher cholesterol later in life, since their bodies need to be challenged with some fat and cholesterol.

Randy: *This sounds symptomatic of questionable nutritional habits, in general. What are the potential health problems that can result from poor childhood nutrition?*

Anne: The potential for obesity is our primary concern, but I've also seen children with hypertension and high cholesterol levels come into my office, caused by an overindulgence of fast food and high-caloric foods and beverages. Diabetes is almost at epidemic levels and children are not exempt. Poor nutrition in childhood can be a risk factor for diabetes or insulin resistance, which can lead to diabetes.

Randy: *If only our kids could discover the beauty of drinking water.*

Anne: If only. That means we have to keep trying to teach them!

Gordon's Tuna Wrap
(Serves 2)

1 4½ ounce can tuna in water, drained
1 teaspoon lite mayonnaise
1 teaspoon plain, non-fat yogurt
2 green onions, sliced

2 soft whole-wheat tortillas
1 handful raw spinach leaves
1 roma tomato, sliced
¼ red apple, sliced

What to Do

1. In a bowl, combine tuna, mayonnaise, and yogurt with finely sliced onions.

2. Warm tortillas in microwave for 10 to 20 seconds and remove. Place on countertop.

3. Spread tuna mixture in center of tortilla. Evenly distribute a few spinach leaves, tomato, and apple slices, keeping the filling away from the edges. Roll up the tortilla and cut wraps in half.

4. Serve immediately or store in refrigerator for tomorrow's lunch.

Nutrients Per Serving
C = 196 • **F** = 3g • **SF** = 1g • **CHO** = 28mg • **CAR** = 28g • **FI** = 4g
P = 19g • **SO** = 0mg • **S** = 5g

Who Is Gordon?
And, Why Is He in Charge of My Tuna Wrap?

Houston is the biggest city in Texas and, with a population of 2.3 million, trails only Chicago, Los Angeles, and New York as the largest city in the United States. With 6 million people living in its surroundings, it ranks as our nation's sixth largest metropolitan area.

So it comes as no surprise that in a population this large and in the midst of a landmass so vast there is one person—Gordon—with the expertise and inspiration to have a tuna wrap named after him.

On the morning of one of our test kitchens, Gordon strolled in all sleepy-eyed and relaxed, hoping like many other local friends of this book that he would soon be enjoying a big batch of free samples.

To everyone's great surprise, Gordon soon turned our culinary world upside down. As Chef Holley was preparing the tuna wrap, Gordon drolly suggested adding a slice of apple. The whole kitchen came to a hushed pause as the chef, the doctor, and the nutritionist all stared at one another. The tension was palpable for a moment until all three nodded in approval. Gordon was obviously moved, and the rest is history. Enjoy your wrap!

Once Upon a Time
When a Bacon, Lettuce, and Tomato Sandwich Was Politically Correct

If you grew up watching television shows like *Ozzie and Harriet*, *The Brady Bunch* or *All in the Family*, you're probably familiar with the traditional BLT sandwich, a cornerstone of the American diet for (way too many) decades. But not any more! It's almost like smoking cigarettes. Most of us have finally figured out that some things are just plain bad for you—like greasy bacon, iceberg lettuce (not bad, just useless), fatty mayo, and the white bread mothers across America always used. We've spared the lovely red tomato from this rude indictment. That's because it's real food, straight from the earth, without any interference, that is, if you buy local or organic. Even though it's a new century and we firmly support progressive and heart healthy eating, we can also appreciate a nice piece of nostalgia. This sandwich is our homage to those bygone days but with a modern, healthy flair.

Without further ado, we present:

Not Your Mama's BLT
(Beets, Leeks, and Tofu)
(Serves 4)

8 ounces roasted beets, sliced
4 leeks, blanched
8 slices of whole-wheat bread or pita

4 ounces extra firm tofu, sliced
2 tablespoons goat cheese
salt/pepper to taste

What to Do

1. After you finish congratulating yourself for even attempting to make this sandwich, begin humming your favorite macrobiotic rock song and place all the ingredients between the two slices of bread, garnish with a copy of *Mother Jones*, and serve.

NOTE: If you have young children, do not answer when they ask you what it is. Quietly leave the room, return to the kitchen, and begin preparing a standard frozen pizza. If you have older children, answer them with something like, "Why can't you be like Gandhi? He ate whatever his mother gave him! And he liked it!" Be firm. Your children will eventually thank you, specifically when they return from the Department of Child and Family Services to report you for snack abuse.

Nutrients Per Serving
$C = 254$ • $F = 5g$ • $SF = 2g$ • $CHO = 4mg$ • $CAR = 45g$ • $FI = 7g$
$P = 11g$ • $SO = 388mg$ • $S = 9g$

All joking aside, this is one tasty sandwich, and its healthy attributes are obvious. But some of you may not be convinced. Chef Holley certainly wasn't. His sous chefs nearly deserted the premises when this item came up in our test kitchen. The idea of beets and tofu occupying the same plate, let alone in a sandwich, was a foreign concept for culinary professionals running a prestigious seafood restaurant. But my collaborator, David Tabatsky, persisted. He claimed that kids in his daughter's school back in New York City were feasting on beets and eating tofu. Well, I guess if they can manage that in the Big Apple, why not here in the Lone Star State? Anne Dubner, our nutritionist, cast the deciding vote, citing the sandwich as a perfectly healthy and delicious dish.

But like I said, some of you may not be convinced. Then again, if you knew some of the other BLT concoctions David came up with, healthy as they might be, you'd be relieved to be eating beets, leeks, and tofu. We mercifully omitted recipes for the following: BLT #2: **B**russel sprouts, **L**ima beans, and **T**urnips. BLT #3: **B**roccoli, **L**ychees, and **T**hyme. Enough said. But this next BLT is a real winner. It may sound goofy, but it's really good. And it's very healthy!

Not Your Mama's BLT #4
(Baked Potato, Lox, and Tomato)
(Serves 1)

1 slice firmly baked potato
1 slice lox (smoked salmon)
1 slice tomato
a splash of lemon juice

salt/pepper to taste
crushed red pepper to taste
lightly toasted whole-wheat hamburger bun (without the hamburger)

What to Do

1. Don't overcook the potato and leave the skin on. Cool. Slice.

2. Add lox (smoked salmon), tomato, lemon juice, and spices. Insert a peace flag into the hamburger bun and serve. Videotape your children's reaction so you have proof that they actually enjoyed this wonderful sandwich.

Nutrients Per Serving
C = 170 • **F** = 4g • **SF** = 1g • **CHO** = 7mg • **CAR** = 25g • **FI** = 2g
P = 9g • **SO** = 348mg • **S** = 4g

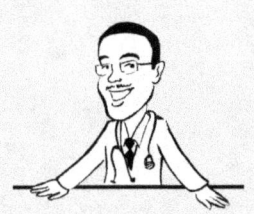

RANDY'S RULES
Get your kids used to drinking water at lunchtime.
It improves taste and has no sugar.

Childhood Nutrition with Randy and Anne

Randy: *What are the biggest mistakes parents make regarding their child's nutrition?*

Anne: Many parents will pressure children into eating all that they serve them, so that they become charter members of the "clean plate club." And all too often, portions are too large, leaving the child feeling overwhelmed.

Randy: *How do we determine the right food dosage for our kids?*

Anne: Start out with smaller portions and allow your child to ask for more if he is still hungry. Never force a child to eat a food that he or she does not want. Give it time, and eventually, he may be willing to try something new.

Randy: *What about the fussy eater?*

Anne: First of all, never use food as a punishment or a reward. This offers the wrong message and can lead to inappropriate eating.

Randy: *Do we let our kids choose what they eat?*

Anne: Parents are often apprehensive about allowing their children to prepare their own meals and snacks, but you will be surprised because when children have the opportunity to prepare food, they are more likely to eat it.

Roasted Chicken Salad on a Bun
(Serves 1)

- 1 multigrain/whole-wheat bun
- 3 ounces Roasted Chicken Salad (below)
- 2 tablespoons jicama, diced
- 1 tablespoon pecans, chopped
- 2 slices of avocado
- 2 slices Roma tomato
- 1 ounce Romaine lettuce, julienned

What to Do

1. Lightly coat a nonstick pan with cooking spray and gently toast the bun on the inside only. Scoop 3 ounces of chicken salad onto the bottom half of the bun. Top with jicama and pecans for some crunch. Add alternating slices of avocado and tomato. Finish with romaine lettuce and the top of the bun.

Nutrients Per Serving
$C = 395 \cdot F = 17g \cdot SF = 3g \cdot CHO = 51mg \cdot CAR = 37g \cdot FI = 6g$
$P = 25g \cdot SO = 2,116mg \cdot S = 8g$

Roasted Chicken Salad
(Serves 4)

- 8 ounces roasted chicken
- 2 tablespoons lite mayonnaise
- 2 tablespoons celery, diced
- salt/pepper to taste
- 2 tablespoons low-fat cream cheese, whipped
- 1 tablespoon Dijon mustard
- 2 tablespoons basil, julienned

What to Do

1. Using leftovers from your chicken dinner, pull chicken meat and add to a large bowl. Combine the rest of the ingredients and mix thoroughly.

Nutrients Per Serving
$C = 516 \cdot F = 17g \cdot SF = 6g \cdot CHO = 210mg \cdot CAR = 13g \cdot FI = 1g$
$P = 76g \cdot SO = 928mg \cdot S = 8g$

This recipe is courtesy of David Cordua from *Artista* in Houston. Some of its ingredients have been adapted for this book.

Box Lunch Bagel
(Serves 1)

1 tablespoon Russian dressing
(lite mayo, ketchup, lemon pepper)
1 mini whole-wheat bagel
1 slice Havarti cheese
½ ounce arugula leaves
1 slice tomato

What to Do

1. Combine mayonnaise, ketchup, and lemon pepper and mix in a bowl.
2. Brush bagel with mixture. Add arugula, tomato, and cheese.
3. Add second half of bagel, close, and place in a baggie.
4. Go to school. Or work. Stop noshing. Go.

Nutrients Per Serving
C = 189 • F = 4g • SF = 2g • CHO = 8mg • CAR = 34g • FI = 6g
P = 8g • SO = 319mg • S = 3g

More Childhood Nutrition with Randy and Anne

Randy: How can parents start educating their kids?

Anne: Begin with the basic Food Guide Pyramid (which can be found online at the American Heart Association website) and build a meal or a snack using at least three of those groups.

Randy: That's what we've done with all the recipes here in the book.

Anne: Absolutely! And having your kids participate can go a long way toward giving them ownership of their own health. Something as simple as a sandwich can be a great accomplishment for a child, leading to positive feelings about food.

Randy: How important is it to establish good eating habits when kids are young?

Anne: When children have positive eating experiences when they are young, it will usually carry on into their teen years and adulthood. But it is just as important for us adults to set good examples with our own healthful food choices so that eating can be viewed as a positive experience, filled with variety, balance, and moderation.

Randy: A balanced diet isn't so hard to accomplish.

Anne: Not at all. Check out the website **www.foodpyramid.gov** for lots of suggestions on balanced meals and snacks.

Tomato Soup Lite
(Serves 4)

1 ounce whole-wheat flour	2½ cups chicken broth, low-sodium
4 tablespoons butter substitute	salt/pepper to taste
2 tablespoons onion, chopped	½ teaspoon white pepper
1 tablespoon green bell pepper	1 tablespoon Roma tomato, diced
½ cup skim milk	½ teaspoon garlic, chopped
1 cup evaporated skim milk	1 teaspoon basil, juilienned
1½ tablespoons tomato paste	1 teaspoon olive oil
14 ounces canned whole tomatoes, peeled	

What to Do

1. In a small nonstick saucepan at medium-high heat, combine flour and 2 tablespoons of butter substitute to make a roux. This will help to thicken the soup. Stir constantly with a spoon until it's toasty brown and a nutty aroma is released. Set aside.

2. Peel an onion and chop it to any size. Chop green bell pepper to any size.

3. In a medium-sized pot, place 2 tablespoons of butter substitute and sauté onion and green bell pepper. Add skim milk, evaporated skim milk, tomato paste, whole tomatoes, and chicken broth. Bring to a boil, whisking constantly. Add salt, pepper, white pepper, and roux, and bring to a boil. Lower heat and continue whisking to avoid sticking or burning. Remove from heat and pass through a fine strainer.

4. In a small bowl, combine fresh, diced roma tomato, garlic, basil, and olive oil to add as a garnish.

NOTE: This soup is perfect for kids who pack a thermos in their lunchboxes.

Nutrients Per Serving
$C = 176 \cdot F = 3g \cdot SF = 1g \cdot CHO = 6mg \cdot CAR = 27g \cdot FI = 2g$
$P = 11g \cdot SO = 429mg \cdot S = 13g$

This recipe is courtesy of David Cordua
from *Amazon Grill* in Houston.
Some of its ingredients have been adapted for this book.

Brown Bag Lunches

The Wright Choice

Five Brown Bag Lunches for Grown-ups

Whether you work at home, in a cubicle, or on the seventy-seventh-floor scaffolding of a new office tower, lunch can be a sacred moment to "stop the madness" if you will. We all need a break in our busy day to stop and refuel—literally. So if you look at it from that perspective—how we need to recharge our body's ability to function at an optimal level, don't you think it makes sense that we eat healthy food? Here are some great ideas, easy to make, that will give you a much needed (and delicious) boost in the middle of your day.

Couscous and Fruit Salad
(Serves 4)

2 cups whole-wheat couscous, cooked
2 teaspoons extra virgin olive oil
1 tablespoon orange juice
1 teaspoon cider vinegar
2 teaspoons shallots, chopped
salt/pepper to taste
1 cup chopped nectarine or plum
1 cup mixed berries
2 teaspoons toasted slivered almonds
canola cooking spray

What to Do

1. Cook couscous according to the specific directions included on the particular brand of couscous you prefer.
2. Whisk oil, orange juice, vinegar, shallots, salt, and pepper in a salad bowl.
3. Lightly coat a small frying pan with cooking spray, and toast almonds on low heat for 2 minutes until toasty brown.
4. Add couscous, fruit, and almonds to bowl. Mint sprig optional. Gently toss and serve.

Nutrients Per Serving
$C = 158$ • $F = 3g$ • $SF = 0g$ • $CHO = 0mg$ • $CAR = 29g$ • $FI = 3g$
$P = 4g$ • $SO = 7mg$ • $S = 9g$

What Is Cous Cous?

A staple for centuries throughout parts of Africa, Europe, and the Middle East, cous cous is a mix of semolina wheat and wheat flour. In some countries, it is made from barley or pearl millet. Its nutritional value is high, and cous cous is considered superior to traditional pastas and rice because of superior glycemic index as well as its vitamin and fat-to-calorie content.

Smoked Salmon Pizza

(Serves 4)

olive oil cooking spray
4 medium pita rounds
¼ pound smoked salmon, thinly sliced
2 tablespoons red onions, chopped
2 tablespoons capers, chopped
¼ cup goat cheese, crumbled
1 tablespoon fresh dill, chopped

What To Do

1. Preheat oven to 350°F. Lightly spray olive oil onto pita bread. Evenly distribute smoked salmon over pita. Sprinkle with red onions, capers, and goat cheese and then add dill. Bake in oven for 5 to 7 minutes.

Nutrients Per Serving

C = 288 • F = 11g • **SF** = 4g • **CHO** = 18mg • **CAR** = 36g • **FI** = 5g
P = 15g • **SO** = 763mg • **S** = 2g

Olive Oil Explained

Why is olive oil so preferred, especially extra virgin cold pressed? It's rich in mono unsaturated fats, one of the most heart healthy fats you can eat. It comes from the highest pick of the olive crop. It's the first press of the olives, meaning it's less processed. And it tastes better! Now, if olive oil is not your favorite, try canola, sunflower, or sesame seed oil. Make sure they are suitable for high-heat cooking.

What's in Your Drawer?

The desk in my office is like a home away from home. I have photographs of my kids, my wife, and a change of clothes in my bottom drawer, just in case I have an emergency at the hospital and need to stay overnight. In my top drawer, I keep a few snacks for those times I start dragging, usually in the late afternoon. As I began working on this book, I realized that even though I was learning to eat better at home and on the road, I still had a drawer full of unhealthy treats in my desk at work.

It was easy to fix. Here's what I keep on hand now, using the recipes right here in this book: homemade power bars and granola, bottled water from home using our own filtered water, and a small plastic bag filled with assorted dried fruit.

Roasted Chicken Chop Salad
(Serves 4)

16 ounces roasted chicken breast, skinless
2 cups romaine lettuce, chopped
⅓ cup cherry tomatoes, halved
2 cups bibb lettuce, chopped
⅓ cup radishes, sliced
sliced croutons

What to Do

1. Preheat oven to 350°F. Place chicken on baking tray, which has been sprayed with canola or sunflower oil. Bake for 10 to 12 minutes or until completely cooked. Remove and cool.

2. Toss all ingredients in a bowl and mix well with Roasted Garlic vinaigrette (recipe below).

NOTE: You may notice a chicken salad in the kids' lunch section. It's a sandwich, easy to make and easy to eat. But while you're preparing the chicken for that recipe you can also prepare the chicken for this salad.

Roasted Garlic Vinaigrette

¼ cup roasted garlic, pureed
2 tablespoons Dijon mustard
2 tablespoons white vinegar
2 teaspoons lemon juice
½ cup lite mayonnaise
2 tablespoons balsamic vinegar
¼ cup water

What to Do

1. Combine all ingredients in a bowl and mix well.

NOTE: Roasted Garlic Vinaigrette was an acrobatic troupe in Detroit in the 1930s.

Nutrients Per Serving
C = 256 • **F** = 8g • **SF** = 2g • **CHO** = 101mg • **CAR** = 7g • **FI** = 1g
P = 37g • **SO** = 171mg • **S** = 1g

Bean Burrito
(Serves 2)

- 4 tablespoons canned pinto beans, drained and rinsed
- ½ teaspoon lemon juice
- 2 tablespoons cheddar cheese
- 1 teaspoon chopped cilantro
- 2 small whole-wheat tortillas
- ¼ avocado, sliced
- salt/pepper to taste

What to Do

1. Place beans and lemon juice in a small bowl and mash with a fork. Mix in cheese and cilantro.
2. Heat the mixture in a microwave for 30 seconds.
3. Spoon the mixture onto the tortillas, roll up, and top with avocado.

Nutrients Per Serving
C = 153 • **F** = 5g • **SF** = 1g • **CHO** = 2mg • **CAR** = 27g • **FI** = 5g
P = 7g • **SO** = 887mg • **S** = 1g

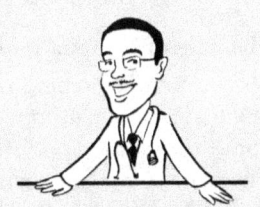

RANDY'S RULES
Drink cool water before a meal.
It improves taste and reduces your appetite.

Texas Caviar
aka
Black Eyed Pea Salad
(Serves 4)

2 15 ounce cans, black-eyed peas, drained
½ cup red onions, chopped
½ cup poblano peppers, diced small
¼ cup red wine vinegar
2 tablespoons cilantro, chopped

salt/pepper to taste
1 cup savoy cabbage, grated
½ cup cherry tomatoes, halved
2 tablespoons garlic, chopped
¼ cup olive oil
1 tablespoon jalapeno, chopped

What to Do

1. Combine all the ingredients and mix well. Marinate for one hour and serve.

Nutrients Per Serving
C = 256 • **F** = 14g • **SF** = 2g • **CHO** = 0mg • **CAR** = 25g • **FI** = 8g
P = 9g • **SO** = 9mg • **S** = 4g

The Tale of Hoppin' John

Chef Holley's recipe, a Lone Star take on old-fashioned rice and beans, was inspired by a culinary tradition with its roots in the southern United States, specifically in South Carolina and Georgia, called Hoppin' John. The origins go way back to the nineteenth century, when soul food took roots in the coastal south, and eating Hoppin' John on New Year's Day was considered good luck. Actually, in some parts of France and Spain it's also considered good luck to eat beans on New Year's.

But who was John, and why was he hoppin'? Legend has it that when the spicy bean dish was brought out, all the kids started hopping around in anticipation. Others say a man named John was so fond of his wife's dish of black-eyed peas and ham hocks that he jumped around town for days, apparently in delight, although he may have simply been moved by the beans. Historians point to the year 1841, when a man named Hoppin' John used to sell a delectable bean dish on the streets of Charleston, South Carolina. Whichever version suits you, we hope you enjoy Chef Holley's dish as much as John once did himself.

Lunch at Home

Lunch Recipes to Enjoy at Home

One reward for working all week or going to school is the chance to relax at home and take time preparing and enjoying meals. Here are some healthy recipes to share with your family on weekends and holidays.

Bow Tie Pasta
(Serves 4)

4 4-ounce boneless, skinless chicken breasts
7 ounces whole-wheat bow tie pasta, cooked
½ cup pitted black olives, chopped
2 tablespoons sun-dried tomatoes, chopped
2 tablespoons white rice vinegar
½ cup roasted peppers, chopped
2 cups raw broccoli florettes
2 tablespoons basil, chopped
1 teaspoon pepper
1 tablespoon olive oil
salt to taste

What to Do

1. Preheat oven to 350°F. Place chicken breasts on a baking pan, which has been sprayed with canola or sunflower oil. Bake for 10 to 12 minutes or until completely cooked. Remove and cool.

2. Bring a large pot of salted water to a boil. Add pasta and cook for 8 to 10 minutes, or until al dente (cooked but still almost kinda crunchy when you bite into it). Place into an ice bath, meaning stay in the kitchen, keep your pants on, and place the cooked noodles into a container with cold water and a few ice cubes. This chilling method keeps the pasta from continuing to cook once it's removed from the heat, ensuring its beautiful texture and ultimate flavor.

3. After you admire your culinary talents, toss in the remaining ingredients and mix well.

4. Store in the frig for several hours before serving. Season with salt and pepper, and just for fun, google "al dente."

Nutrients Per Serving
C = 445 • **F** = 11g • **SF** = 2g • **CHO** = 96mg • **CAR** = 43g • **FI** = 5g
P = 44g • **SO** = 340mg • **S** = 4g

Somebody's Shrimp Boil
(Serves 4)

¼ cup crab boil
1 teaspoon sea salt
4 new potatoes, peeled and cooked
12 button or small oyster mushrooms
1 pound raw jumbo shrimp, with shell

2 pieces yellow corn on the cob
2 whole garlic cloves, peeled
2 cups diced onions
6 lemons with peel, halved

What to Do

1. Fill large pot with 6 quarts of water and bring to a boil.
2. Add crab boil and salt.
3. Add remaining ingredients, except shrimp, and return to a boil. Cook 10 minutes or until potatoes are cooked, but still firm.
4. Add shrimp and simmer for 7 to 10 minutes. Remove from pot and strain. Serve with cocktail sauce (see below) and garnish with lemons.

NOTE: Shrimp is higher in cholesterol than some other seafood, but it's lower in saturated fat and has the benefits of omega-3 fatty acids, which are heart healthy.

Nutrients Per Serving
C = 243 • **F** = 3g • **SF** = 1g • **CHO** = 172g • **CAR** = 27g • **FI** = 4g
P = 33g • **SO** = 760mg • **S** = 6g

Traditional Cocktail Sauce

1 tablespoon prepared horseradish
1 teaspoon fresh lemon juice
¼ teaspoon fresh ground black pepper

1 cup ketchup
3 dashes Tabasco sauce

What to Do

In a large bowl, combine all of the ingredients and stir well.
By the way, a dash of Tabasco means a simple shake of the bottle – one dash equals one shake. No more. No less.

Nutrients Per Serving
C = 66 • **F** = 0g • **SF** = 0g • **CHO** = 0mg • **CAR** = 17g • **FI** = 1g
P = 1g • **SO** = 740mg • **S** = 7g

Chilled Asparagus Soup
(Serves 4)

2 pounds asparagus
½ cup onion, chopped
1 tablespoon garlic, chopped
1 cup leeks, chopped
6 cups low-sodium chicken stock

1 potato, large, diced
4 ounces spinach, fresh or frozen
plain non-fat yogurt
salt/pepper to taste
vegetable chips

What to Do

TIP: Buy pencil asparagus (the long skinny ones) whenever possible. If you can find only the thicker version, make sure you cut off the brown and woody parts on the bottom.

1. With either type of asparagus you purchase, cut off the top 2 to 3 inches, which are your asparagus spears. Keep the rest for later. Blanch the spears in boiling water for 5 to 6 minutes. Drain thoroughly. Rinse with cold water and set aside.

2. In a medium, nonstick saucepan, combine onions, asparagus (the lower parts), garlic, and leeks. Sauté over low heat for 5 to 6 minutes.

3. Add stock and potatoes and simmer for 10 minutes or until potatoes are tender. Add spinach. Remove from heat for 2 to 3 minutes.

4. Puree soup in a food processor or blender until smooth. Chill well.

Note: If your soup is a bit too thick, you can thin it with some chicken stock. (Just to remind you, there are 2,300 mg of sodium in one teaspoon of salt. This recipe has less than that.)

5. Serve each bowl with a swirl of non-fat yogurt, asparagus spears, and vegetable chips.

Nutrients Per Serving
C = 119 • **F** = 1g • **SF** = 0g • **CHO** = 1mg • **CAR** = 7g • **FI** = 7g
P = 8g • **SO** = 977mg • **S** = 7g

What Are Healthy Vegetable Chips?

Just as potato chips have become as varied as breakfast cereals, so, it seems, have vegetable chips. Supermarkets and health food stores offer many different brands and styles. You don't even have to look very hard to find non-fat and low-fat versions. The trick is to look a little harder and try to find one that is relatively low in sodium. Good luck!

Roasted Sweet Potato Soup
(Serves 4)

2 cups pureed sweet potatoes
(you'll need 3 to 5 medium sweet potatoes, depending on size)
1 tablespoon vegetable oil
1 cup leeks, small, diced
1 cup yellow onions, small, diced
1 teaspoon fresh garlic, minced
48 ounces chicken stock (low sodium, fat-free)
salt/pepper to taste
brown sugar to taste
2 tablespoons hot sauce
1 tablespoon Worcestershire sauce
¼ teaspoon nutmeg
½ teaspoon sage
2 teaspoons cinnamon

What to Do

1. Preheat oven to 350°F. Bake sweet potatoes for 45 minutes or until tender. Remove from oven and cool to room temperature. Peel potatoes and discard the skin. Slice into large chunks.

2. In a pot over medium heat, add oil, leeks, onions, and garlic and cook for 6 to 8 minutes. Add sweet potatoes, stock, and remaining ingredients (except salt, pepper, brown sugar) and bring to a boil. Lower heat and simmer for 15 to 20 minutes, stirring occasionally. Remove from heat and let cool.

3. Puree the soup in blender for 1 minute or until smooth. Return to pot and slowly bring to a boil. Thin to desired consistency with chicken stock.

4. Season with salt, pepper, and brown sugar, as preferred.

Nutrients Per Serving
C = 210 • **F** = 5g • **SF** = 1g • **CHO** = 1mg • **CAR** = 40g • **FI** = 3g
P = 4g • **SO** = 1138mg • **S** = 27g

What is a Chipton?

Imagine a potato chip and a crouton. Chipton. Get it? Okay, how do I make one?

Combine Quinoa (half cup), millet (half cup). Add a little bit of garlic, parsley, salt and pepper, cumin, turmeric, and olive oil.

Mix together, press flat into a cookie sheet and bake for 45 minutes. Cool. Eat. Enjoy! (Thanks, Rachel.)

Deconstructed Hard Boiled Egg Salad
(Serves 4)

6 egg whites
cooking spray
½ teaspoon lemon juice
½ cup lite mayonnaise
1 tablespoon celery, minced

1 tablespoon onion, minced
1 teaspoon Dijon mustard
1 teaspoon sweet relish
16 stone wheat crackers
1 teaspoon chives, chopped

What to Do

1. Separate egg whites from egg yolks. The reason we use only egg whites in this recipe is because the egg yolks contain all the cholesterol and we are concerned about keeping those levels down. So just adjust your eyes to white eggs!

2. Over medium heat, lightly coat a nonstick frying pan with cooking spray and cook egg whites for 1 to 2 minutes. When they become solid, remove from heat and chop. Set aside.

3. In a bowl, add lemon juice, mayonnaise, celery, onions, mustard, and relish and mix well to make the sauce.

4. Serve in three bowls (eggs, sauce, crackers) for people to construct their own dish. Or you can assemble by putting the sauce on a cracker with egg on top and add chives to garnish.

Nutrients Per Serving
C = 145 • **F** = 4g • **SF** = 0g • **CHO** = 0g • **CAR** = 21g • **FI** = 2g
P = 7g • **SO** = 571mg • **S** = 7g

Your Choice of Crackers

With your health in mind, it's vital that you pay attention to your choice of crackers. We recommend stoned wheat. If you think you may be overdoing it on your cracker intake, try scooping up that egg salad with a stalk of celery.

What Do I Do with Those Egg Yolks?

Since egg yolks are full of cholesterol (and fat) we don't recommend eating them on a day-to-day basis. However, once in a while, they come in handy for doing some old-fashioned baking at home. If that's your hobby, store the yolks in the freezer for one of those rainy days when you're home baking with your kids.

Turkey Sloppy Joe
(Serves 6)

canola cooking spray
1 cup finely chopped onion
½ cup green bell pepper, chopped
¾ pound ground lean turkey
1 tablespoon chili powder
1 teaspoon fresh oregano

1 14.5-ounce can tomato sauce
¼ cup ketchup
2 tablespoons tomato paste
1 tablespoon Worcestershire sauce
½ teaspoon dried red pepper
6 whole-wheat hamburger buns

What to Do

1. Lightly spray canola oil in a large pan and bring to a medium heat. Sautee onions and peppers until soft. Add ground turkey and cook until no longer pink. Stir in chili powder, red pepper, and oregano and cook for 1 minute.

2. Add tomato sauce, ketchup, tomato paste and Worcestershire sauce. Cook for 15 to 20 minutes on low heat. Remove from heat and let sit for 5 minutes.

3. Divide equally between 6 buns and serve.

NOTE: You may notice that these portions are somewhat smaller. This is intentional, in keeping with the concept of meat as a side dish, or at least a smaller sized main course.

Nutrients Per Serving
$C = 144$ • $F = 5g$ • $SF = 1g$ • $CHO = 45mg$ • $CAR = 14g$ • $FI = 3g$
$P = 12g$ • $SO = 636mg$ • $S = 6g$

A Vegan Alternative

Most supermarkets today are selling vegan products, including sausages, bacons, and various other vegetarian "meats." Most of them have a zero fat content and a high concentration of protein, a perfect combination for a heart healthy diet.

When you compare the price to various cuts of meat you will be pleasantly surprised. You'll also end up feeling better when you begin eating less red meat!

Pork or Shrimp Stir-Fry
(Serves 4)

SAUCE
- ¼ cup soy sauce, low-sodium
- ¼ cup water
- 2 tablespoons Hoisin
- 1 tablespoon sesame oil
- 2 teaspoons fish sauce
- 1 tablespoon serrano, chopped

- 1 cup broccoli florettes, blanched, sliced
- 1 cup asparagus, blanched, sliced
- 1 cup baby carrots, blanched, sliced
- 12 ounces whole-wheat spaghetti, cooked
- cooking spray
- 1 tablespoon vegetable oil
- 2 tablespoons green scallions, thinly sliced
- 8 ounces pork, thinly sliced, or shrimp
- 1 tablespoon garlic, chopped
- 1 tablespoon ginger, chopped
- 1 cup shitake mushrooms, sliced
- ¼ cup snow peas, thinly sliced
- 1 tablespoon cilantro, chopped

What to Do

1. To make sauce: In a bowl, add soy sauce, water, Hoisin, sesame oil, fish sauce, and serrano. Mix well and set aside.

2. Blanche broccoli, asparagus, and carrots. Cut into 2-inch slices and set aside.

3. Heat large pot of water to boil. Cook pasta until al dente. Drain. Lightly coat pasta with vegetable spray. Set aside.

4. In a wok or large sauté pan, add oil over high heat. Add pork (or shrimp), garlic, and ginger, and sauté for 3 to 4 minutes, stirring constantly.

5. Add mushrooms and snow peas, and sauté for 1 more minute.

6. Add broccoli, asparagus, carrots, and sauce and simmer for 5 to 6 minutes or until sauce has thickened. Remove from heat. Add cilantro and scallions and mix together.

7. Lay warm pasta onto a plate and top with stir-fry.

Nutrients Per Serving
C = 394 • F = 14g • SF = 3g • CHO = 67mg • CAR = 36g • FI = 5g
P = 32g • SO = 963mg • S = 4g

Nutrients Per Serving (Shrimp)
C = 259 • F = 8g • SF = 1g • CHO = 43mg • CAR = 38g • FI = 5g
P = 13g • SO = 1,090mg • S = 5g

NOTE: While pork is higher in protein, shrimp is lower in calories, fat, and cholesterol. Then again, shrimp is higher in sodium. Maybe tofu sounds good.

Dinner!

Picnic Dinners and Weekend Feasts

Between work and school and family affairs, we are a busy bunch, trying to cram as much as we can into a limited amount of time. It's when we're in a hurry that we often make the worst choices for our health, especially when it comes to food. But it doesn't have to be that way. Whether it's those spring and summer evenings when you rush home to eat dinner so you can make it to your son's or daughter's Little League game on time, or those long weekend and holiday drives to your in-laws when it would be great to have your own food on hand instead of stopping at a fast-food joint on the highway, you have control of your choices! Here are five alternatives for any number of these occasions.

Almost Meatless Chili
(Serves 4)

- 1 cup red onions, chopped
- 2 tablespoons fresh garlic, chopped
- ½ cup poblano peppers, chopped
- 1 tablespoon serrano peppers, chopped
- 2 tablespoons olive oil
- 4 cups vegetable stock (no MSG)
- 4 ounces turkey bacon, cooked and chopped
- 12 ounces nonalcoholic beer
- 1 teaspoon chili powder
- 2 cups red kidney beans, cooked
- 2 cups black beans, cooked
- ½ teaspoon ground cumin
- 1 lime, freshly squeezed
- 2 tablespoons cilantro, chopped

What to Do

1. In a large saucepot, sauté onions, garlic, peppers, and olive oil over medium-high heat for 2 to 3 minutes.

2. Add vegetable stock, bacon, beer, chili powder, beans, and cumin and simmer for 20 to 25 minutes, stirring occasionally.

3. Add lime and cilantro and simmer for an additional 5 minutes. Remove from heat and serve with brown rice or low-fat tortilla chips.

Nutrients Per Serving
C = 416 • **F** = 14g • **SF** = 3g • **CHO** = 25mg • **CAR** = 53g • **FI** = 17g
P = 22g • **SO** = 652mg • **S** =7g

Leg of Lamb with Ratatouille
(Serves 6)

Lamb

2 tablespoons garlic, chopped
2 tablespoons Creole mustard
1½ tablespoons rosemary, chopped

1 tablespoon Creole seasoning
2 pounds lamb, uncooked

What to Do

1. Preheat oven to 300°F.

2. In a bowl, combine garlic, mustard, rosemary, and Creole seasoning and mix well. Rub lamb thoroughly with seasoning mixture and marinate for 1 to 3 hours (the longer the better).

3. Roast lamb for 60 to 90 minutes until the lamb is cooked to your preference.

TIP: Make sure to select a brand of Creole seasoning that's low in sodium.

Nutrients Per Serving
C = 329 • **F** = 14g • **SF** = 4g • **CHO** = 113mg • **CAR** = 12mg • **FI** = 3g
P = 37g • **SO** = 397mg • **S** = 4g

Ratatouille

1 tablespoon olive oil
1 cup zucchini, diced large
1 cup yellow squash, diced large
1 cup red onion, julienne
¼ cup garlic, sliced
1 cup eggplant, diced large
1 cup button mushrooms, halved

½ cup green peppers, julienned
½ cup red peppers, julienned
¼ cup red wine (optional)
1 cup cherry tomatoes, halved
1 tablespoon fresh basil, chopped
1 teaspoon fresh oregano, chopped

What to Do

1. In a sauté pan, over medium-high heat, add oil, zucchini, squash, and red onions and sauté for 3 to 5 minutes. Add garlic, eggplant, mushrooms, and peppers and continue to sauté for 3 more minutes. Add wine and continue cooking for 2 more minutes. Add tomatoes, basil, and oregano and remove from heat.

Johnny Cakes with Jerk Chicken
(Serves 4)

Johnny Cakes
(Mini-pancakes)

1 cup cornmeal
½ cup whole-wheat flour
1 teaspoon baking powder
½ teaspoon salt
cooking spray

¼ cup egg substitute
¼ cup skim milk
¼ cup water
¼ cup corn, frozen (optional)

What to Do

NOTE: First of all, don't panic because there are two grams of saturated fats in this recipe (or a lot of sodium). Once in a while, it's okay. Just watch your diet the rest of the day by avoiding excess amounts of fat and salt.

Now, for the cakes themselves:

1. In a bowl, combine all the dry ingredients and mix well. In another bowl, combine the wet ingredients (eggs, milk, and water) and mix well. Put the two together and mix well.

2. Using a griddle (preferred) or nonstick frying pan over medium heat, coat lightly with cooking spray and pour in individual (2-ounce) portions of the mixture. When bubbles appear, flip and continue cooking until golden brown. Remove and serve.

Who's Johnny and Is He Really a Jerk?

Johnny, who this recipe was named after, was a pioneer back in the eighteenth century who journeyed through the Northeast in search of something else to eat besides cornmeal, a staple of many diets during that era. It wasn't that Johnny didn't like cornmeal; it's just that he grew bored eating it three times a day.

In modern times, Johnny Cakes is known as a rather sullen gangster on the hit TV show *The Sopranos*. Mr. Cakes has no known association with the cornmeal industry; however, he is known to enjoy a well-made meal.

And just to set the record straight, the expression "jerk chicken" comes from the Caribbean, which means that Johnny is definitely not a jerk!

Jerk Chicken
(Serves 4)

1 whole chicken, skinless, cut into 8 pieces	1 cup onions, julienned
2 tablespoons jerk seasoning	¼ cup green onions, thinly sliced
1 tablespoon curry powder	¼ cup sliced garlic, thinly sliced
2 teaspoons red cracked pepper	1 cup non-fat, chicken stock (no MSG)
1 lemon, thinly sliced	salt/pepper to taste
2 cups green peppers, julienned	

What to Do

1. Preheat oven to 350°F. Cut chicken into 8 pieces. Remove skin.

2. In a small bowl, combine jerk seasoning, curry powder, and red cracked pepper and mix well.

3. Sprinkle and rub chicken pieces well with seasonings. Marinate for 3 hours in a casserole dish.

4. Place sliced lemons on top and sprinkle green peppers, onions, garlic, and green onions. Add 1 cup of chicken stock, cover with foil, and bake for 45 to 50 minutes.

**Nutrients Per Serving
(Cakes and Chicken)**

C = 495 • **F** = 11g • **SF** = 3g • **CHO** = 90mg • **CAR** = 58g • **FI** = 8g
P = 41g • **SO** = 922mg • **S** = 6g

Who Is Julienne and What Is She Doing in My Recipe?

All this talk about another woman in your kitchen might be making you nervous, but it's simply a French word for "sliced." There they go again, those funny French people, making trouble in America! Just kidding. Thank God for French food. And thanks to whoever invented slicing stuff. Yea! No more choking. Good idea.

Blackened Catfish Over Sautéed Spinach Topped with Mango Papaya Salsa

(Serves 4)

4 6-ounce catfish portions
cooking spray
Creole seasoning
2 teaspoons vegetable oil
1 teaspoon garlic, chopped
¼ cup red onions, julienned
8 ounces spinach

What to Do

1. Coat fish well on both sides with cooking spray. Sprinkle Creole seasoning on both sides of fish and rub in well.

2. Preheat cast-iron skillet until very hot. Cook fish for 2 to 3 minutes per side until blackened and fully cooked.

3. In a separate sauté pan, over medium heat, add oil, garlic, and onions and sauté for 2 minutes. Add spinach and sauté until it is completely wilted. Season with salt and pepper to taste.

Mango Papaya Salsa

1 tablespoon fresh mint, diced
1 cup mango, diced small
2 tablespoons olive oil
1 tablespoon red bell peppers, diced small
1 tablespoon green bell peppers, diced small
1 cup papaya, diced small
1 tablespoon fresh basil, chopped
2 tablespoons rice wine vinegar
honey

What to Do

Mix all ingredients in a bowl. Add honey as needed and serve.

Nutrients Per Serving
(Fish and Salsa)

C = 215 • **F** = 7g • **SF** = 1g • **CHO** = 66mg • **CAR** = 18g • **FI** = 3g
P = 21g • **SO** = 215mg • **S** = 13g

Ginger Tofu Fried Rice
(Serves 4)

2 cups jasmine rice, cooked
olive oil cooking spray
14 ounces firm or extra firm tofu, cubed
1 teaspoon sesame oil
½ cup red onions, chopped
1 tablespoon garlic, chopped
1 cup snow peas, sliced
1 tablespoon fresh ginger, chopped
¼ cup red bell peppers, chopped
2 egg whites
2 tablespoons low-sodium soy sauce

What to Do

1. Cook rice according to package directions.

TIP: If you have a rice cooker, you're guaranteed perfect rice. When using a saucepot, here's a tip for cooking jasmine rice. Once you've followed the box's directions and your rice is finished, remove from heat and cover the pot with plastic wrap. Let it sit for 5 minutes. This will help the rice become flaky.

2. In a large, nonstick skillet or wok over medium-high heat, coat with olive oil spray. Sauté tofu carefully for 2 to 3 minutes until light brown. Remove from pan. Set aside.

3. In the same pan, over medium-high heat, add sesame oil, onions, garlic, snow peas, ginger, and red peppers, and sauté for 3 to 4 minutes.

4. Add cooked rice and cook for 3 minutes, stirring occasionally.

5. Stir in egg whites and cook for one minute until mixed well.

6. Add soy sauce and tofu and cook for an additional minute, stirring gently so tofu stays intact.

Nutrients Per Serving
C = 258 • **F** = 2g • **SF** = 0g • **CHO** = 0mg • **CAR** = 46g • **FI** = 2g
P = 13g • **SO** = 417mg • **S** = 3g

Meat As a Side Dish

Are you afraid of withdrawal symptoms if you give up red meat and start eating tofu? If all that healthy food is making you pine for a steak, go ahead and have some! But just cut down on your portions. If, for example, your son is a rapidly growing, active teenager, adding a four-ounce steak to the tofu fried rice is not such a bad idea.

You, on the other hand, perhaps somewhere in your "middle ages," should prepare only half of that portion. Think of that steak as a side dish—a few bites to satisfy your urge for meat and keep you from overindulging next time you go out to eat.

Chicken Ahuacatl (Awacottle)
(Serves 2)

1 7 ounce chicken breast, boneless, skinless,
1 tablespoon extra virgin olive oil
2 to 3 ounces Avocado Mousse (see recipe below)

2 ounces Pineapple Jicama Escabeche (see recipe next page)
salt/pepper to taste
½ teaspoon smoked paprika
cilantro leaf

What to Do

1. Season chicken with olive oil, salt, and pepper and grill on medium heat for 4 minutes on each side. Once chicken is fully cooked, finish with smoked paprika. **2.** Place Avocado Mousse on plate and put chicken on top. Garnish with escabeche and cilantro leaf.

Please Note: This is a heart healthy way to eat chicken. The fats may sound high at first, but you can relax because these fats are polyunsaturated and mostly monounsaturated fats, both of which are good for your arteries.

Nutrients Per Serving
C = 276 • **F** = 14g • **SF** = 3g • CHO = 84g • **CAR** = 5g • **FI** = 2g
P = 32g • **SO** = 389mg • **S** = 2g

Avocado Mousse
(Serves 4)

garlic, 1 clove
jalapeño (pinch) as needed
1 tablespoon cilantro leaves, base stems removed
salt (pinch)

1 tablespoon white wine vinegar
1 avocado
1 ounce water
3 ounces non-fat Greek yogurt
1 tablespoon extra virgin olive oil

What to Do

1. In a blender, combine garlic, jalapeño, cilantro, salt, vinegar, avocado, and water. Add more water if needed to loosen up the mixture.
2. Add Greek yogurt and blend. Slowly pour in olive oil in a stream until emulsified.

Nutrients Per Serving
C = 132 • **F** = 11g • **SF** = 2g • CHO = 0g • **CAR** = 6g • **FI** = 3g
P = 4g • **SO** = 8mg • **S** = 2g

Pineapple Jicama Escabeche
(Serves 4)

½ cup pineapple, diced
¼ cup red onion, diced
1 teaspoon jalapeño, minced
2 tablespoons lime juice
½ cup jicama, diced
¼ cup tomato, diced
2 tablespoons cilantro, chopped
½ teaspoon salt

What to Do
1. Dice all ingredients into ¼-inch pieces.
2. In a medium-sized bowl, combine all ingredients. Each serving will be just over two ounces.

Nutrients Per Serving
$C = 22$ • $F = 0g$ • $SF = 0g$ • $CHO = 0g$ • $CAR = 6g$ • $FI = 1g$
$P = 32g$ • $SO = 293mg$ • $S = 4g$

These recipes are courtesy of David Cordua
from *Americas* in Houston.
Some of its ingredients have been adapted for this book.

Jasmine Jambalaya
(Serves 6)

- 1 cup jasmine rice, uncooked
- cooking spray
- 1 pound boneless chicken breast, cubed
- 1 tablespoon vegetable oil
- 1 cup onions, chopped
- ½ cup green peppers, chopped
- ½ cup celery, chopped
- 3 garlic cloves, smashed
- 3 cups fat-free chicken broth
- 1 tablespoon hot sauce
- 1 tablespoon Worcestershire sauce
- 1 tablespoon creole seasoning
- ¼ cup green onions, thinly sliced
- ½ pound turkey sausage, sliced
- ½ cup canned diced tomatoes, strained

What To Do

1. Cook rice following directions on package.

TIP: See recipe for Ginger Tofu Fried Rice on page 337.

2. Preheat oven to 350°F. Place chicken breasts on a baking pan that has been sprayed with canola or sunflower oil. Bake for 10 to 15 minutes or until completely cooked. Remove and cool.

3. In a large pot, over medium-high heat, sauté onions, green peppers, celery, and garlic in vegetable oil for 4 to 5 minutes, or until onions are tender. Add remaining ingredients (hot sauce of your choice!) and mix well. Cover and simmer for 15 to 20 minutes.

Nutrients Per Serving

C = 340 • **F** = 10g • **SF** = 3g • **CHO** = 74mg • **CAR** = 31g • **FI** = 2g
P = 30g • **SO** = 752mg • **S** = 3g

The Rice Cooker Method
aka
Idiot Proofing Your Kitchen

The idiot proofing is named after me. Using a rice cooker is so easy even a five-year-old can do it. Not that we recommend young children playing with appliances. Just making a point about how easy it is for an adult to use a rice cooker as an effective method for cooking things like Jasmine Jambalaya, the One Pot Breakfast, and even Mac 'n' Cheese, whichever version you choose to make.

Salmon in Foil
(Serves 4)

4 6-ounce portions Atlantic salmon fillets
salt/pepper to taste
8 ounces asparagus, blanched
1 each red, yellow, green bell peppers
8 ounces shitake mushrooms, sliced
1 teaspoon sesame oil
1 tablespoon rice vinegar
¼ cup olive oil
1 teaspoon sesame seeds
1 tablespoon low-sodium soy sauce

What to Do

1. Preheat oven to 400°F. Season the salmon fillets with salt and pepper.

2. Blanch asparagus (see procedure in recipe for One Pot Breakfast, page 298).

3. Cut 4 square shaped pieces of aluminum foil, large enough to hold each portion of fish and vegetables. Place the fish on one side of the foil.

4. Cut peppers into circular pieces (rings) and lay them down, one by one, color by color, on top of the fish. Place asparagus inside the rings and sprinkle mushrooms on top of them. If this is confusing, check the website for a photo. If you're on a remote island without a computer, you can mix the ingredients in almost any way and the flavors will still come through when you cook the fish. But the rings are cool!

5. In a small bowl, combine oil, rice vinegar, sesame oil, and soy sauce. Mix sauce well. Add 1 tablespoon of this mixture over each piece of fish. Sprinkle sesame seeds on top.

6. Cut another large sheet of foil (the same size as the first) and place on top of each piece of fish. Pinch the top and bottom pieces of foil together (with the fish inside) and seal the edges. Make sure they're tightly sealed! Place on a baking sheet and bake for 10 to 15 minutes, depending on the thickness of the fillets.

Nutrients Per Serving
C = 387 • **F** = 24g • **SF** = 3g • **CHO** = 78mg • **CAR** = 9g • **FI** = 3g
P = 31g • **SO** = 209mg • **S** = 3g

Mac 'n' Cheese:
The Good, the Bad, and the Inedible

Legend has it that Mac 'n' Cheese was invented in the aftermath of World War I when building supplies, specifically caulking materials, were seriously lacking. A fellow named Vinnie, who lived with his wife, Shirley, in a blue-collar section of Chicago, came up with the idea one day at lunchtime while working a construction site on the south side of town. Shirley had packed him a hefty portion of macaroni pasta and as Vinnie sat there, looking at his coworker munching on a chunk of cheese and staring at the cracks in the walls that desperately needed caulking, something suddenly inspired him.

He came back the next day with a solution in his lunchbox. As his co-workers looked on in dismay, Vinnie proceeded to patch up all the cracks with a concoction he'd whipped up at home the night before.

"Whaddaya doin' Vin?" his partner, Nuncio, asked him.

"Watch this, my friend," Vinnie replied, as he spread out his homemade paste on all the walls.

"What is that stuff?" Johnny Knuckles called out. "It smells weird!"

"Hey! Respect. It's macaroni 'n' cheese!" Vinnie cried out. "And it works! The cracks are fixed. Come here and look."

So Nuncio and Johnny K. did just that. Before long, they had eaten most of Vinnie's handiwork. However, the point had been made. Combining macaroni noodles and a hefty cheese sauce had potential. Soon enough, Vinnie and Shirley were in business, making homemade mac 'n' cheese and selling it house to house and block by block, all over Chicago. That was back in the day, when they used homemade pasta and unadulterated cheese. It tasted good but it was pretty bad for you: high in the wrong kinds of fat, high in cholesterol, and very low down on the heart healthy scale.

Then things got worse. Food manufacturers, who had been packaging highly processed foods with increasing frequency, decided to co-op the mac 'n' cheese world by making an instant version. All one had to do was cook the noodles and then simply pour in a dry version of something they referred to as cheese. Like I said, things went from bad to worse. Trouble is, they made it so cheap and quick to prepare that it became too darn attractive to pass up. Housewives and homemakers began buying boxes by the dozen. Soon enough, they were feeding their families dinner-in-a-box at least two or three times a week. It's no wonder that children began putting on too much weight, started developing stomach problems, and faced increasing difficulties with their digestion. Hard to believe people are still eating this stuff! It's downright inedible!

So let's swing to the good side of mac 'n' cheese. Let's consider a recipe to make Michelle Obama smile and, more important, something that will help our kids get healthier.

You can begin with your choice of pasta. Why not use whole-wheat elbow noodles or corn shells? How about vegetable spirals or rice noodles? The options are huge, so experiment and have a mac 'n' cheese fest at home. That should include some healthy choices for the dairy side, beginning with organic, non-fat or skim milk, butter substitute, and some smart cheese choices. Try low-fat cheddar, low-fat Swiss, or even better, you can choose from an array of cheeses made from soy, rice, or almonds, all of which are healthier than their dairy cousins. Once again, experiment.

In fact, why stop with the traditional categories? You can add yellow squash, leftover chicken (shredded), or tofu, or all three. Most kids won't even realize some of it is in the mix. Some, though, may applaud you for it. Congratulations! Your mac 'n' cheese is now in the "good" category.

Nana's Leftovers

Culinary anthropologists report that the "modern leftover age" began in 1945 with the invention of Tupperware by Earl Tupper. These plastic containers made it possible for an entire generation of homemakers to preserve just about anything and completely redefined the concept of the expiration date.

In all seriousness, it is vital that you pay attention to a food's expiration date, especially with meat and dairy items, and take care not to keep leftovers too long. If you do, it's certainly at your own risk, as history so aptly shows.

For example, according to the Institute of Useless Information, the record for the longest sustained consumption of leftovers was set by a woman named Lillian Ungerleider, who was living in a small village in Hungary back in 1914. After cooking a traditional pot of

Hungarian goulash, Mrs. Ungerleider made it last for an unbelievable 171 days, adding in a steady stream of vegetables, assorted meats, shoes, sweat, and a pinch of resentment for her neighbors in Bulgaria. It goes without saying that Mrs. Ungerleider's goulash became a bit distasteful by day 171, when she decided enough was enough.

All joking aside, keep your food properly refrigerated.

And in case your mother hadn't already shown you by example, leftovers work wonders for all sorts of uses: lunches on the go, picnics in the park, snacks in the backseat, and dinners on those days when you just don't have the time or energy to deal with any of these fantastic recipes.

Snacks

Snacks

Gosh, if it weren't for snacks, I might hardly eat on some days. That may be an embarrassing admission but more important, it's a dangerous habit to get into, for anyone! If you're busy like me, you may miss a meal a few times during the week and snacking may be your only way to keep food coming in while you're on the go. I'm not judging whether that's a good thing or not. I'm simply acknowledging the reality for many people out there, hustling to work, going nonstop all day, and rushing home to take care of their kids, their lawn, and their community before plopping into bed for an all too short night's sleep, before doing it all over again the next day. Unfortunately for too many folks out there, this is the American way.

Chef Bobo reminded me that "fast food" can be made at home where you can control what's going into it. For example, chicken nuggets can be made with fresh chicken breast cut to resemble nuggets and then breaded and roasted in the oven. He adds, "Fresh food, which doesn't have to cost more, does require more personal time, but that's a good investment for the future and it is definitely fiscally responsible."

That's right. It all starts at home, not just with major meals, but at snack time, too, whether they're eaten in your kitchen, in your car, at your desk, or at the soccer field. If you're forced to eat like this on some days, you can at least eat something cost-effective and healthy!

SnackSpeak with Randy and Anne

Randy: *What are the best snacks for kids after school that won't ruin their dinner?*

Anne: Be sure that you monitor your children's after-school snacks. Some healthy choices include raw fruit cut into cubes and skewered onto pretzel sticks, veggies with a low-fat dip or salsa, a smoothie made with yogurt and frozen fruit, or the old stand-by, "ants on a log," celery filled with peanut butter and raisins placed on top. Again, see how creative your child can be, choosing healthful foods as a base for snacks.

Randy: *Sounds like good advice for parents, too.*

Anne: Of course! And the recipes you have in the book are terrific examples of great tasting, healthy food for kids and their parents.

Randy: *I'm hungry.*

Anne: Me, too.

What To Do When Children Invade Your House

Your twelve-year-old just decided to invite the chess team home after school. And his sister is suddenly hosting a playdate for four of her friends. Out of the blue, you've got eleven kids in your house, a five-year-old to look after, dogs to walk, and a project proposal due tomorrow morning on your boss's desk. But it's 4 p.m., meaning snack time at kid central! You've got to get your act together and feed those cute little you-know-whats.

Start with popcorn. It's quick, painless, and the mess is manageable. But beware. Popcorn is high in fiber and naturally low in calories and fat, but most manufacturers of the microwavable treat still manage to stuff 250 calories and more than 15 grams of fat into each bag. Some food companies promote popcorn as cholesterol-free and a good source of fiber. They also want you to believe that popcorn is the healthy choice when it comes to snack foods, whether you're in the movie theater or at home. Ha ha. Look closely and you'll see that commercial popcorn is largely UNhealthy!

But don't despair. There are a few good products out there with just a few grams of fat per serving and fewer calories. Read the labels and you'll see. To impress your daughter and her friends, try this: using a simple spray bottle (like you may have for plants), fill it with some olive oil and spray the popcorn just once or twice to give it a minimally light coating. The kernels will absorb the olive oil as you shake it up in a bag. Then sprinkle Parmesan cheese and a pinch of sea salt over it. Shake it again. To jazz it up even more, add a bit of cayenne. It packs a little kick!

If you've got kids with a bigger hunger, try mini-muffin pizzas with whole-wheat English muffins, marinara sauce, and low-fat mozzarella cheese. You may even add your child's favorite vegetable. Top that off with a non-fat granola parfait, easy and quick to throw together, and perfectly healthy. If you are going to run the risk of compromising your children's appetite for dinner, you may as well fill them up with healthy food.

Don't worry. We haven't forgotten about you. After the kids are asleep and you've cleaned up around the house (or not!), it's time you had a small indulgence of your own, at least once in a while. There's a treat on the next page we're sure you'll enjoy.

Whole-Wheat Bagel Surprise
A Late Night "Adult" Snack
(Serves 1)

1 shot brandy (1 ounce)
4 slices peaches, fresh or frozen
2 teaspoons tofu-based cream cheese

1 whole-wheat mini-bagel
½ teaspoon cinnamon
pinch of nutmeg

What to Do

1. First of all, don't down the brandy (yet).
2. In a small dish, pour brandy and soak peaches in it for 20 minutes.
3. Spread cream cheese on bagel.
4. Add peaches, cinnamon, and nutmeg.
5. Leftover brandy optional.

Nutrients Per Serving

C = 357 • **F** = 4g • **SF** = 1g • **CHO** = 0g • **CAR** = 58g • **FI** = 7g
P = 7g • **SO** = 386mg • **S** = 24g

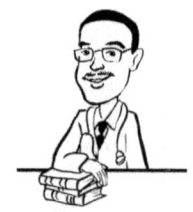

THE WRIGHT ADVICE

Speaking of alcohol, moderation is key.
A glass of red wine is considered heart healthy,
but making it a daily habit is not recommended.
Check with your doctor to see what's best for you.

Salads!

The Wright Choice

The Fastest Salads in America

It's a Tuesday, you're in a hurry, with no time to figure out any tremendous new dinner ideas (you don't even want to negotiate these recipes), and you definitely want a night free of washing pots and pans. At the same time, you feel that it's important to put a healthy meal on the table for your family, and you're determined to do so. Bravo! Once you have the ingredients on hand, any of the following salads (and dressings) can be made in less than five minutes by a certified member of the adult species. These recipes are intended to produce side dishes, not main courses, but with a few leftovers on hand, you'll have a terrific and nutritious meal you can be proud to serve. You can even enjoy it yourself!

Spinach Salad
(Serves 4)

2 ounces turkey bacon
8 ounces spinach
¼ cup red onions, julliene
¼ cup pecans, halved and roasted
¼ cup mushrooms, sliced

What to Do

1. In a nonstick pan, sauté bacon over medium heat until crispy. Blot on a paper towel and chop.

2. In a bowl, toss spinach, bacon, red onions, pecans, and mushrooms. Add Honey-Citrus Mustard Dressing (recipe on page 356) and serve immediately.

Nutrients Per Serving
C = 96 • **F** = 8g • **SF** = 1g • **CHO** = 13mg • **CAR** = 4g • **FI** = 2g
P = 4g **2** • **SO** = 260mg • **S** = 1g

Waldorf with a Twist
(Serves 2)

¼ cup beets, diced
cooking spray
2 tablespoons walnuts, toasted

¼ cup apples, diced
¼ cup grapes, quartered
¼ cup arugula
¼ cup celery hearts

Dressing

¼ cup lite mayonnaise
1 tablespoon honey

1 teaspoon lemon juice
salt/pepper to taste

What to Do

1. Preheat oven to 325°F. Lightly spray the beets with cooking spray. Wrap in aluminum foil and place on a tray in the oven for 45 to 60 minutes.

2. Add walnuts to the tray when you are 5 minutes away from removing the beets. Toast them for the remaining time. Let beets cool and dice.

3. In a bowl, add mayonnaise, honey, and lemon juice, and mix well. Season to taste. Add remaining ingredients and mix well. Use walnuts as a garnish.

Nutrients Per Serving
C = 195 • **F** = 15g • **SF** = 1g • **CHO** = 10mg • **CAR** = 18g • **FI** = 1g
P = 2g • **SO** = 263mg • **S** = 13g

Do You Love the Beets?

Maybe you thought the twist to the Waldorf salad was the arugula lettuce. Kind of. But it's the beets that make this dish unique. Mixed in as they are with all the other ingredients, it could be a great way to introduce your kids to this very healthy vegetable.

In case you missed it back in the Lunch section, we have another recipe using beets. Check out Not Your Mama's BLT on page 310.

Organic Quinoa Salad
(Serves 2)

- 1 ounce spring mixed greens
- 1 teaspoon extra virgin olive oil
- 1 teaspoon lime juice
- 1 cup cooked Quinoa (recipe next page)
- 1 tablespoon heart of palm, diced
- 1 tablespoon red bell pepper, diced
- ½ teaspoon basil, chopped
- 1 tablespoon tomato, diced
- 1 tablespoon poblano pepper, roasted and diced
- 4 ounces grilled chicken, skinless
- 1 teaspoon Cotija cheese, grated
- ½ teaspoon cilantro, chopped

What to Do

1. Toss mixed greens in 1 teaspoon of olive oil and 1 teaspoon of lime juice and place in the center of a large salad bowl.

2. Lay a large row of quinoa down across the center of the bowl over the mixed greens. Arrange rows of each vegetable on either side, saving slices of grilled chicken for last.

3. Garnish quinoa with Cotija cheese, cilantro, and basil.

Nutrients Per Serving

C = 480 • **F** = 17g • **SF** = 3g • **CHO** = 99mg • **CAR** = 40g • **FI** = 7g
P = 44g • **SO** = 181mg • **S** = 1g

What Is Quinoa?

It's actually not a grain. It is the seed of the Chenopodium or Goosfoot plant, with more than 120 species, and it's been growing in South America for thousands of years. Quinoa (pronounced keen-wa) is high in protein, calcium, and iron and is a good source of Vitamin E and many of the B vitamins. For those with certain allergies to wheat, you'll be glad to know that quinoa is gluten free. It cooks easily and quickly and complements salads, fish, and chicken. It works well as an alternative to rice and you can add foods to it to make a nice risotto. Search the Internet for lots of additional information.

Quinoa
(Serves 2)

½ tablespoon onion, diced
½ tablespoon carrot, diced
½ tablespoon celery, diced
salt to taste

½ tablespoon olive oil
½ cup dry quinoa
1½ cups water

What to Do

1. In a small sauté pot, begin to sauté onion, carrot, and celery in olive oil until translucent. Add quinoa and toast thoroughly (5 to 8 minutes) until grain reaches a deep, roasted color and releases a toasted aroma.

2. Add water and salt and heat to a rolling boil. Lower heat to a simmer. Once liquid is almost completely dry and there are holes where bubbles had formed, turn off heat and cover the pot with its lid or use aluminum foil. Allow to rest covered for 15 to 20 minutes or until all liquid is absorbed and quinoa is cooked through.

3. Spread over a cookie sheet and cool in the fridge to stop from overcooking.

Nutrients Per Serving
C = 191 • **F** = 6g • **SF** = 1g • **CHO** = 0mg • **CAR** = 30g • **FI** = 3g
P = 6g • **SO** = 11mg • **S** = 0g

Please Note

With this recipe, you'll be making the equivalent of two servings of quinoa. You can use what's left over with any number of other foods.

This recipe is courtesy of David Cordua from *Americas* in Houston.

Some of its ingredients have been adapted for this book.

Panzanella Salad
(Serves 4)

- 12 sweet cherry tomatoes, halved
- ¼ cup English cucumbers, thinly sliced
- ¼ cup red onion, thinly sliced
- ¼ cup kalamata olives, sliced
- 2 cups croutons
- salt/pepper to taste
- ½ cup goat cheese
- 1 teaspoon extra virgin olive oil
- 4 celery hearts
- 2 teaspoons fresh basil, chopped

What to Do

1. In a large salad bowl, combine the tomatoes, cucumbers, onions, olives, croutons, and basil. Toss well, season with salt and pepper.

2. To serve, divide the salad among four bowls. Top with goat cheese and drizzle with olive oil. Garnish with celery hearts and basil.

3. Serve with Sweet Onion Vinaigrette (below).

Nutrients Per Serving
C = 209 • **F** = 13g • **SF** = 4g • **CHO** = 8mg • **CAR** = 19g • **FI** = 3g
P = 6g • **SO** = 432mg • **S** = 1g

Sweet Onion Vinaigrette

- ¼ cup sweet onions, diced
- ¼ cup olive oil
- ½ tablespoon Dijon mustard
- 2 tablespoons rice wine vinegar
- 2 teaspoons fresh basil, chopped

What to Do

1. In a bowl, combine all ingredients and mix well.

Nutrients Per Serving
C = 125 • **F** = 14g • **SF** = 2g • **CHO** = 0mg • **CAR** = 1g • **FI** = 0g
P = 0g • **SO** = 48mg • **S** = 0g

Southwestern Cobb Salad

(Serves 4)

1 12-pound pork tenderloin, roasted and sliced
salt/pepper to taste
6 cups romaine lettuce, chopped
¼ cup red onions, julienne
½ cup black beans, canned, rinsed
½ cup corn, fresh or frozen
½ cup avocado, large diced
1 ounce tortilla strips

What to Do

1. Preheat oven to 350°F. Season pork with salt and pepper and place on baking tray in the oven for 30 to 45 minutes, until pork is thoroughly cooked.

2. Remove from oven and cool to room temperature before slicing.

3. In a large serving bowl, put the lettuce in and top with red onions.

4. Arrange beans, corn, pork, and avocado in separate rows next to the romaine.

5. Drizzle dressing as needed. Gently toss to combine all ingredients before serving.

6. Garnish with tortilla strips.

NOTE: This is a traditional salad, meant to be served tableside. Make a video and send to YouTube.

Dressing

1 tablespoon chipotle peppers in a dobo sauce (can be purchased as described)
2 teaspoons lime juice
½ cup lite mayonnaise
2 tablespoons fresh cilantro, chopped
¼ cup water
salt/pepper to taste

What to Do

1. In a bowl, combine ingredients and mix well.

Nutrients Per Serving
(Salad and Dressing)

C = 327 • **F** = 18g • **SF** = 3g • **CHO** = 55mg • **CAR** = 22g • **FI** = 7g
P = 21g • **SO** = 319mg • **S** = 2g

Salad Dressings
Heart Healthy and Homemade

These are fun to make with your kids, economical, and heart healthy. Aprons recommended.

Warning! Do not like these too much! Don't drink the dressing! Each recipe serves 4 to 6 people, depending on how much you use. We recommend you be modest in your dosage. These dressings can also be interchanged with the salads, depending on your preferences.

Poppy Seed Vinaigrette

½ cup plain, non-fat yogurt
1 tablespoon rice wine vinegar
2 teaspoons mint, chopped
2 tablespoons olive oil
2 tablespoons poppy seeds
1 tablespoon honey

What to Do

1. Play that new CD you just bought. Combine all ingredients in a bowl and mix well.

NOTE: Poppy Seed Vinaigrette was a garage band in the 1980s in Milwaukee.

Nutrients Per Serving
C = 92 • F = 7g • SF = 1g • CHO = 0mg • CAR = 6g • FI = 0g
P = 2g • SO = 19mg • S = 5g

Honey-Citrus Mustard Dressing

1 tablespoon Creole mustard
1 teaspoon lime juice, freshly squeezed
1 teaspoon lemon juice, freshly squeezed
1 teaspoon fresh orange juice
¼ cup olive oil
1 teaspoon honey

What to Do

1. In a bowl, combine all ingredients and mix well. Don't overdo the honey!

Nutrients Per Serving
C = 99 • F = 11g • SF = 1g • CHO = 0mg • CAR = 1g • FI = 0g
P = 0g • SO = 39mg • S = 0g

Dad's Super Sunday Grill

The Wright Choice

Dad's Super Sunday Grill

Even though it's 2011 and times change, it's still mostly moms who are buying books and cooking dinner. But it's a different story come Sundays, when dads bust out their silly aprons and start up the barbecue. And, unfortunately, many dads still cook up some bad news, like fatty steaks, ribs, and chicken in all their unhealthy skin.

Can we take a time-out and reboot the grill?

Our intrepid chef, Mark Holley, has concocted some terrific healthy recipes for dads to execute and for everyone else to enjoy. Have a great weekend!

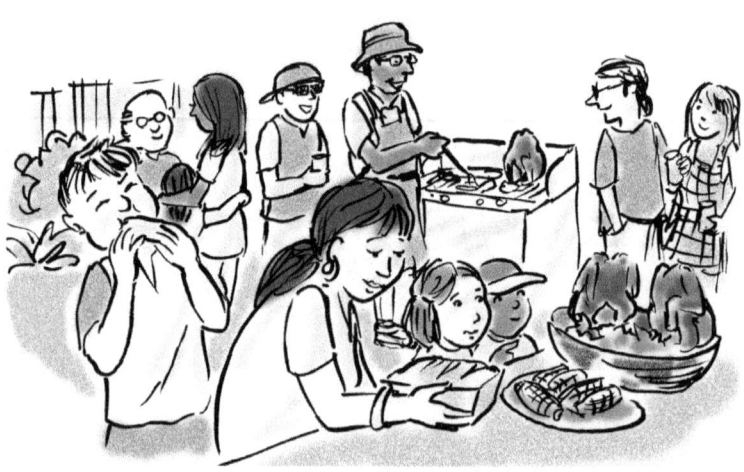

Charcoal versus Gas

Speaking of grills, everyone has his preference, and who are we to tell a man what grill works best for him? Who are we? We're from Texas, that's who! Born to barbecue! In the Lone Star State, babies learn to grill before they can even walk.

But Chef Holley knows a thing or two about grilling, and here are his tips on the great controversy: charcoal versus gas.

Charcoal: It's labor intensive, and it spews carcinogens. One also needs to know how to burn off the charcoal before you start putting raw food on it. But the advantage is flavor—especially with wood chips.

Gas: It's clean and needs less maintenance. You just turn it on and it goes, providing a more even distribution of heat, with no carcinogens. As for flavor, you can use an attachment with wood chips, offering you the best of both worlds.

Gas grills may be more expensive but our survey of one says they're well worth it.

FYI

When it comes to food, mason jars come in handy. I've recently discovered how useful they are as shakers and storage containers for salad dressings. Put all the ingredients into a jar, seal it well, and shake it up. It often works better than mixing the dressing by hand.

Cajun Meatloaf Burger
(Serves 6)

1½ pounds extra lean ground beef
1 tablespoon fresh garlic cloves, chopped
½ cup mushrooms, chopped
¼ cup rolled oats
¼ cup tomato sauce
2 tablespoons cajun seasoning
1 cup red onions, chopped
¼ cup poblano peppers, chopped
¼ cup egg substitute
½ teaspoon chili powder
1 tablespoon Worcestershire sauce
1 teaspoon ground oregano

What to Do

1. Combine all ingredients into a large bowl. Mix well (by hand) until thoroughly combined.

2. Shape into patties and place on the grill.

Nutrients Per Serving
C = 242 • F = 11g • SF = 4g • CHO = 41mg • CAR = 8g • FI = 1g
P = 26g • SO = 658mg • S = 2g

The Bun Wars

Remember my friend back in the hospital? He bought a big, greasy hospital burger and then skipped the bun, thinking he was doing the healthy thing by avoiding the carbs in the bun. Well, he did avoid eating a chunk of unnecessary, unhealthy white bread, but scarfing down a cheap hamburger didn't do him any favors.

Our menu offers you the chance not only to eat a healthy hamburger; we're offering you the option to have your burger with a healthy dose of carbs that comes from whole-wheat bread, be it a bun, pita bread, or an English muffin.

Grilled BBQ Veggies
(Serves 4)

1 tablespoon olive oil
2 tablespoons low-sodium soy sauce
2 tablespoons garlic, chopped
1 each tricolored bell peppers (red, yellow, and green), quartered
1 pound asparagus
1 red onion, quartered
1 yellow squash, quartered
8 ounces portobello mushrooms

What to Do

1. Heat grill as your directions indicate.

2. Place grill screen (recommended) on grill and coat with oil. Aluminum foil will do if you don't have a screen.

3. In a small mixing bowl, combine olive oil, soy sauce, and garlic, and mix well. Coat vegetables with mixture and place on grill screen until browned and tender. Turn as needed. Grill time is approximately 5 minutes per side but will vary depending on thickness and type of vegetable.

Nutrients Per Serving
C = 133 • F = 4g • SF = 1g • CHO= 0g • CAR = 21g • FI = 7g
P = 7g • SO = 264g • S = 9g

Lifesaving Barbecue Etiquette

For those of you who will be attending someone else's barbecue as a guest, please note that while we highly recommend indulging your host's hospitality with good manners of your own, that doesn't have to guarantee that you indulge in every food they have to offer.

For example, if the burgers down the street are being served only on white bread buns, go ahead and break your rules on eating white bread. It's not only the polite thing to do; it could keep your shirt clean. But when you are hosting, you can supply your guests with whole-wheat buns.

Beer Butt Chicken
(Serves 4)

1 whole chicken, skinless
2 teaspoons olive oil
2 tablespoons rosemary, chopped
2 tablespoons roasted garlic (see recipe)
2 tablespoons lemon juice, freshly squeezed
1 can beer
salt/pepper to taste

What to Do

1. In a bowl, combine all ingredients except chicken to make garlic paste.

2. Remove skin from chicken. Rub the chicken inside and out with garlic paste. Marinate for at least 3 hours, but preferably overnight.

3. Heat the grill. Open can of beer. Lower the chicken onto the can, placing the can into the internal cavity of the bird. Place the chicken so that legs become a tripod, holding the chicken upright.

4. Place on grill and cook until done. Take photos!

Nutrients Per Serving
C = 155 • **F** = 4g • **SF** = 1g • **CHO** = 63mg • **CAR** = 3g • **FI** = 1g
P = 25g • **SO** = 58mg • **S** = 0g

(FOR DAD'S EYES ONLY)

Alcohol evaporates. Use light beer. You can also use alcohol-free beer. Can't find alcohol-free beer in a can? Put it in an empty cola can. Better still, make that a diet cola can. Even better, use an empty can of organic soda. Your kids (and your wife) will never know you're drinking nonalcoholic beer.

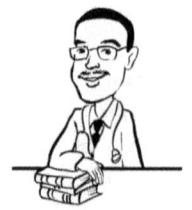

THE WRIGHT ADVICE

Speaking of beer or wine or whatever you may be partaking of, do it in moderation, especially in front of your kids.

Grilled Flank Steak
(Serves 4)

4 5-ounce raw flank steaks
1½ cup Chimichurri Sauce (see below)
1 teaspoon kosher salt
fresh ground pepper

What to Do

1. Place steaks in a large baking dish and coat them with the Chimichurri sauce on both sides. Cover and marinate in the refrigerator for 2 hours.

2. Preheat the grill to high. Remove steaks from the refrigerator 30 minutes before grilling.

3. Remove steaks from the marinade and season with salt and pepper. Grill for 6 to 7 minutes on one side, turn over, and continue grilling for 5 to 6 minutes to reach a temperature of medium.

4. Remove from the grill, let rest for 10 minutes, and serve with remaining chimichurri on the side.

Chimichurri Sauce

2 tablespoons cilantro, minced
1½ tablespoons fresh oregano, minced
2 limes, juiced
½ teaspoon kosher salt
4 tablespoons parsley, minced
⅓ cup Spanish olive oil
8 garlic cloves, minced
1 teaspoon fresh ground pepper

What to Do

1. Combine all ingredients in a bowl and season with salt and pepper.

2. Divide the chimichurri between 2 bowls. Use half as a marinade and half as the finishing sauce.

Nutrients Per Serving
C = 396 • **F** = 28g • **SF** = 7g • **CHO** = 76mg • **CAR** = 4g • **FI** = 1g
P = 32g • **SO** = 569mg • **S** = 1g

Nana's Leftovers

Many of the ingredients in these recipes mix and match together and make great candidates for exciting leftovers. In these challenging economic times, it behooves all of us to be thoughtful about how we recycle our meals. Today's omelet may have been yesterday's banquet, and Sunday's barbecue can make an excellent goulash or stew on Monday. Use your imagination to save money and create new recipes!

What About Dessert?

Some (if not all) of you may be looking here for dessert recipes, but you won't find them. That's because, as much as we also enjoy our sweets, we think it's best to focus on the main part of our daily diets. Besides, we've included a number of sweet foods that can also satisfy those cravings. We recommend that you serve fresh fruit as much as possible.

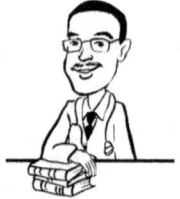

THE WRIGHT ADVICE
Dessert is NOT Mandatory!!!
Eating a healthy meal doesn't give you permission to indulge by eating an UNhealthy dessert.

Shhh! Don't Tell the Kids

Sometimes, deceiving your children is not only allowed; it's recommended. Imagine you're making brownies—your kids' favorite dessert—and you add some zucchini or yams or tofu to boost their nutritional value. Do your kids really need to know? That's the kind of deception we're referring to. You can do the same thing with oatmeal cookies and a number of other desserts. Check our website for new tips on healthy desserts. www.TheWrightChoiceRx.com

Sugar Substitutes

In our quest to get healthier, we look to replace the foods that we know are bad for us. For example, when we discuss desserts (who doesn't?), we're almost always talking about sugar. We already know that white sugar—any sugar, in fact—can be harmful, especially when overused, which it is, all too often by most of us. So we figure that using honey instead of sugar takes care of part of that problem. Wrong. Honey is not automatically a "healthy" replacement for sugar. Both of them contain fructose and glucose, two elements we should minimize in our diets.

Imagine you want to substitute one spoonful of honey in your tea for that scoop of sugar you normally use. One tablespoon of sugar contains 46 calories. An equivalent amount of honey has 64 calories. Granted, honey is a bit more intense and we need less of it to do its sweetening thing, but most people don't control the dosage and end up adding unnecessary calories. So while honey is preferable to white sugar, it has issues of its own. That's why we've minimized its inclusion in these recipes, suggesting agave syrup as a somewhat healthier alternative, and suggesting you use it minimally—see "drizzle."

The solution is to lessen your need for sweetening, gradually, until you can do away with it altogether or merely use a pinch—really, we mean literally a pinch. In the meantime, avoid artificial sweeteners. When you're talking about food, doesn't the word "artificial" seem out of place? Rather than risk your health with any of those, try Stevia, a very sweet herb from South America, or Xylitol, also known as birch sugar, which is very low on the glycemic index and can be healthy for you in small doses.

Moderation is the key. In fact, sometimes abstinence is the safest bet.

The Power of Good Habits

As we've discussed throughout this book, it's up to you to develop good habits and make a daily commitment to sticking with them. When in doubt, following the American Heart Association recommendations is a safe bet. On the next few pages, you'll find a three-week menu planner to help make life at home a bit easier.

A Three-Week Menu

The Wright Choice

Week 1

	Breakfast	**Lunch**	**Dinner**
MONDAY	Cherry Oatmeal and non-fat milk/yogurt	Peanut Butter Tea Sandwiches Cous Cous/Fruit Salad	Johnny Cakes Jerk Chicken Waldorf Twist
TUESDAY	Power Bar and Smoothie	Gordon's Tuna Wrap (kids) or Salmon Pizza (adults)	Ginger Tofu Fried Rice Panzanella Salad
WEDNESDAY	Granola Smoothie	Not Your Mama's BLT or Roasted Chicken Chop Salad	Somebody's Shrimp and Asparagus Soup
THURSDAY	Crepe Ambrosia	Trail Mix Cracker and/or Texas Caviar	Almost Meatless Chili Waldorf Twist
FRIDAY	Cherry Oatmeal non-fat milk/yogurt	Box Lunch Bagel or Bean Burrito	Salmon in Foil and Spinach Salad
SATURDAY	Mediterranean Latkes or Quesadilla Margarita	Frittata and Tomato Soup	Chicken Ahuacatl and Quinoa Salad
SUNDAY	Smoked Salmon Omelet or Turkey Pita	Turkey Pita and/or Waldorf Twist	Flank Steak and Grilled Veggies

Week 2

	Breakfast	Lunch	Dinner
MONDAY	Power Bar and Smoothie	Not Your Mama's BLT #4	Blackened Catfish and Quinoa Salad
TUESDAY	Cherry Oatmeal and non-fat milk/yogurt	Roasted Chicken Salad on Bun and/or Couscous Fruit Salad	Jasmine Jambalaya and Spinach Salad
WEDNESDAY	Granola and Smoothie	Box Lunch Bagel or Bean Burrito	Meatless Chili and Waldorf Twist
THURSDAY	Cherry Oatmeal and non-fat milk/yogurt	Gordon's Tuna Wrap and Texas Caviar	Stir Fry and Cobb Salad
FRIDAY	Buckwheat Blueberry Pancakes and non-fat milk/yogurt	Peanut Butter Tea Sandwiches or Smoked Salmon Pizza	Turkey Sloppy Joe and Panzanella Salad
SATURDAY	Crepe Ambrosia and/or Frittata	Quesadilla Margarita and Tomato Soup	Leg of Lamb Baked Potato and Spinach Salad
SUNDAY	One Pot Breakfast or Smoked Salmon Omelet	Mediterranean Latkes and Sweet Potato Soup	Beer Butt Chicken and Pasta and Grilled Veggies

The Wright Choice

Week 3

	Breakfast	Lunch	Dinner
MONDAY	Cherry Oatmeal and non-fat milk/yogurt	Trail Mix Crackers and Tomato Soup or Roasted Chicken Chop Salad	Jasmine Jambalaya and Panzanella Salad
TUESDAY	Granola and Smoothie	Gordon's Tuna Wrap and/or Texas Caviar	Turkey Sloppy Joe and Spinach Salad
WEDNESDAY	Crepe Ambrosia and non-fat milk/yogurt	Not Your Mama's BLT and/or Cous Cous/Fruit Salad	Somebody's Shrimp and Panzanella Salad
THURSDAY	Power Bar and Smoothie	Peanut Butter Tea Sandwiches or Bean Burrito	Salmon in Foil Baked Sweet Potato and Spinach Salad
FRIDAY	Cherry Oatmeal and non-fat milk/yogurt	Box Lunch Bagel and/or Smoked Salmon Pizza	Ginger Tofu Fried Rice and Cobb Salad
SATURDAY	Buckwheat Blueberry Pancakes and non-fat milk/yogurt	Bow Tie Pasta and/or Deconstructed Egg Salad	Chicken Ahuacatl and Quinoa Salad
SUNDAY	Frittata and Fresh fruit	Mediterranean Latkes and Tomato Soup	Cajun Burger and Grilled Veggies

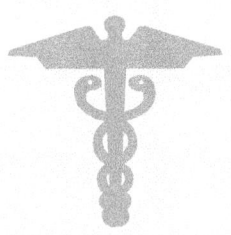

The Wright Reminders

Plan meals ahead and stick to your plan.

Eat as a family whenever possible.

Limit alcohol consumption.

Be creative.

Bon Appétit!

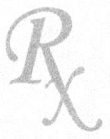

CHAPTER 14

The Family Training Zone

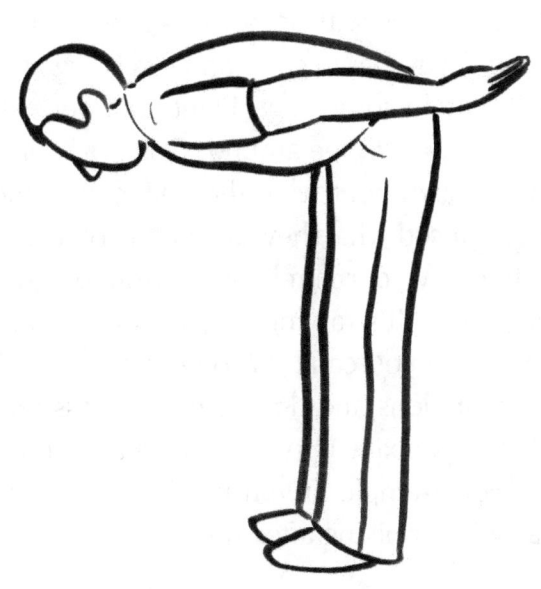

An Active Family Is a Happy Family

Most people think that cancer is the number one killer in America. It's not. Cardiovascular disease holds that distinction, and in most cases it is directly related to insufficient exercise and unhealthy eating. It's not rocket science. Physical activity leads to good health, which leads to happy families. The government's latest health recommendations for adults suggest at least 30 minutes a day of moderate physical activity, such as brisk walking or hiking. Or, if you are able, something more vigorous, like jogging, swimming, or biking. As far as your cardiovascular health is concerned, your body doesn't care what type of exercise you perform; it just wants you to move!

For those of you with some grass around your house, you sure don't have far to go to find some engaging physical activity. Build something. Plant a garden. Play with the dogs. Throw a frisbee around. Go for a walk and talk with your family about what they hear, see, and smell. You'd be surprised what they say when you actually take the time to enjoy your immediate surroundings.

What's that? It's raining? Try an umbrella! There's really no reason you can't do *something* every day. You might get ambitious and double your fitness time a few days a week by mixing up your routine and adding some activities. For example, if you jog 30 minutes a day try adding a swim or biking afterward.

The Family Training Zone

STOP!

EXERCISE BREAK!

Reading about exercise is all fine and good, but if that's all you do you're in big trouble.

Time to practice what we are preaching (that's if you haven't already been doing the exercise breaks in all the previous chapters).

Last time, you did 25 minutes. Or did you?

This time, let's make it 30.

That way, when you get to the next (and last) chapter, you won't be surprised.

The Good Old-Fashioned Body Test

How many push-ups and sit-ups can you do? Check the chart below to see where you stand.

Push-Up Test (Men)

Age	17–19	20–29	30–39	40–49	50–59	60–65
Excellent	> 56	> 47	> 41	> 34	> 31	> 30
Good	47–56	39–47	34–41	28–34	25–31	24–30
Above average	35–47	30–39	25–34	21–28	18–25	17–24
Average	19–34	17–29	13–24	11–20	9–17	6–16
Below average	11–18	10–16	8–12	6–10	5–8	3–5
Poor	4–10	4–9	2–7	1–5	1–4	1–2
Very Poor	< 4	< 4	< 2	0	0	0

Push-Up Test (Women)

Age	17–19	20–29	30–39	40–49	50–59	60–65
Excellent	> 35	> 36	> 37	> 31	> 25	> 23
Good	27–35	30–36	30–37	25–31	21–25	19–23
Above Average	21–27	23–30	22–30	18–25	15–21	13–19
Average	11–20	12–22	10–21	8–17	7–14	5–12
Below average	6–10	7–11	5–9	4–7	3–6	2–4
Poor	2–5	2–6	1–4	1–3	1–2	1
Very Poor	0–1	0–1	0	0	0	0

Source: Adapted from Golding, et al. (1986). *The Y's way to physical fitness* (3rd ed.)

While Jack LaLanne could have outdone us all we owe it to ourselves (and our loved ones) to be around in good health for as long as possible. Adults should also do muscle

The Family Training Zone

strengthening activities at a moderate or high-intensity level two or more days a week, including exercises for the chest, back, shoulders, upper legs, hips, abdomen, and lower legs. You can include free weights or machines (neither of which are free), resistance bands (same), or calisthenics that use body weight, such as push-ups, pull-ups, and sit-ups (all free). Those of you with backyards may already be carrying heavy loads or doing the kind of gardening that requires heavy lifting.

It's simple, really. Walk. Walk fast. Jog. Run. Jump up and down (if you can). Push, pull, lift, and carry. The point is: Be active!

For example, next time you take out the garbage at night for the next day morning pick up, carry the can or bag around for 5 to 10 minutes before setting it down. Bend over and touch your toes 10 times. Do 50 jumping jacks. Some squats. Breath in the night air—at least a few feet away from the garbage. Drop and do 10 push-ups. If it's dark out, don't worry; no one will see you. That's helpful, especially if you get inspired and decide to do the whole routine again. Who wins? You and your improved health.

And your dog, too, if you have one. According to a study conducted by the University of Missouri-Columbia participants, none of whom were regular walkers, who walked their dog 20 minutes a day, 5 days a week, for 50 weeks lost an average of 14 pounds. It goes without saying that their dogs benefited, as well.

Now, what about your kids, watching their nutty mom or dad from the living room window, running around the yard with a garbage can? If they're old enough, have them join in so they can exercise along with you. But don't wait for them to figure that out. Why don't you initiate the fun? You'd be doing everyone a big favor. In fact, research proves the point.

The National Institute of Health recommends that children and adolescents should engage in an hour or more of moderately intense to vigorous aerobic physical activity each day. That's daily, not weekly, and should involve bone-strengthening movement, such as running, and muscle-strengthening activity, such as tug-of-war or modified sit-ups and push-ups. If your kids are old enough, you can stop pampering them and make them do their sit-ups and push-ups the old-fashioned way! Once again, you'll be doing them a favor!

If it is raining and you're stuck inside, try this. Instead of opting for playing a family board game, try some indoor sports. Pick your favorites that you enjoy playing together on whatever media program you may have at home. If you can't decide what to play, toss your ideas into a hat and have someone choose. Go from there! For those of you who don't use your television for these things, you can be creative without any electronics. Your kids are probably in the midst of school and studies. Need to work on math facts or spelling words? Make a relay race to get the homework done. Place various obstacle points throughout the house (or yard). Starting at one end, have someone read you the word or math fact, then if you get the answer run to the next obstacle. Keep going until you get to the end. Then do it backward! If you get one wrong, go to the beginning. Either way, you and your kids will be up and moving, exercising your bodies, as well as your minds.

Tips to Get Fit

1. Be honest about your current condition and create realistic expectations. Too much, too fast may cause injuries. If you are new to regular exercise, approach it carefully. Begin with low-impact activities. If you are overweight or just facing an expiration date on your joints, try swimming, cycling, or walking. Thinking you will look better after a few days is kind of silly and can lead to overtraining, burnout, or injury. Go slow and be steady. And make sure your family members follow the same advice.

2. Be committed and have fun. Work out for at least 30 minutes daily, interspersed throughout the day, if necessary. Do what you like, not what someone on TV says is right for you. Get your spouse and your kids to join in, whenever possible. And don't forget: Warm Up! Cool Down!

3. Don't settle for easy goals. Even if you're really new to exercising, challenge yourself! Choose activities that are appropriate for your current fitness level and gradually increase the intensity and duration. If you stick with it, you will see results.

4. Develop a Total Fitness Plan. Include aerobic conditioning, weight lifting, and flexibility training. Aerobic movement develops stamina and improves your cardiovascular system. Weight-bearing exercise can slow down osteoporosis. Increased flexibility will prevent injuries and help you sleep better. Keep track of your progress by writing things down.

5. Consider fitness as your new lifestyle. Integrate walks, hikes, or group sports into your daily life. You can work up a good sweat without going to the gym. Hint: Try the stairs instead of the elevator.

Please Note: If you have pre-existing medical conditions consult a health care provider before beginning an exercise program.

Calorie Burn

Everybody wants to burn calories. But as you discovered in Chapter 9, it's vital that you keep track of what you eat and what you burn. That math is vital for losing weight and maintaining good health.

Did you know that kissing burns 25 calories per hour? If only we all made time for that each day (and had a partner we wanted to kiss that much!). Think about that when you compute how many calories you might be burning doing any of the activities in the following chart. Besides sleeping, sitting, and standing, how many of these do you maintain for an hour on any given day? How vigorously do you do any of them? No matter how you answer (honestly, we hope), you can always improve. In fact, if you're single, getting out of the house to exercise may increase your chance of meeting someone you'd like to kiss for an hour.

Activity	Calories Burned per Hour	Activity Level
Sleeping	55	Low
Eating	85	Low
Sitting	85	Low
Standing	100	Low
Driving	110	Low
Office work	140	Low
Housework	160+	Moderate
Golf (with no cart)	180	Moderate
Dancing (ballroom)	260	Moderate
Walking (3 mph)	280	Moderate
Tennis	350+	Moderate
Aerobics	450+	Moderate
Jogging (5 mph)	500	High
Gardening (active)	500	High
Swimming (active)	500+	High
Hiking	500+	High
Rowing	550+	High
Biking (studio)	650	High

Calculating Heart Rate

This is a math formula but not an exact science. However, it will provide a good starting point for your cardio work. 220 − RHR − AGE = THR.

220 minus your Resting Heart Rate (RHR) minus your age equals the base number used to calculate your Training Heart Rate (THR). To determine your RHR, take your pulse on three mornings for a full 60 seconds before you get out of bed. The average of those three days will be used in the math formula. For example, 220 − RHR of 70 − 48 years old = 102; this number will be used in the next calculation for determining your THR.

Appropriate heart rate for training depends on your fitness level when you start this program. If you have not been exercising at all (or had a fitness program in the past but have not kept it up), you need to start at a lower percentage than people who have been training.

For example, using the number 102 from above, calculate your THR at 60 percent of your Maximum Heart Rate (MHR). The formula is as follows: 102 x .60 = 61.2 + RHR (70) added back in for a total of 131.2 as your THR. After you've trained at this rate for a while and built some endurance, you can start moving incrementally to a higher THR of perhaps 80 percent, or 151.6. You might work at the 131 range for three minutes, then work at the higher rate for one minute, then back to 131.

Set a realistic time frame and specific goals for your fitness program. "I want to lose some weight" is too vague. "I want to lose 20 pounds in six months" is a specific goal. Make a commitment to change your lifestyle, not just something you're going to do for three months and then go back to your old habits. I'm also a big believer in a rewards system as you reach your goals. If your goal is to get everyone in your family involved in a fitness program, then maybe a family trip can be the reward for achieving those goals.

The Hidden Gym in Your Home

If you have a ball in your house or one in the garage, then you possess a universe of possibilities. Do you have stairs? Perfect. Even one will do for some things. Most everyone has at least a few things lying around that can be used for exercise. You'd be surprised what you forgot you have in your garage or basement. For example, what about that jump rope you bought years ago, thinking you'd use it after you gave birth to your son, but then you got too busy and too tired and too good at making up excuses not to use it? It's time to find that thing and dust it off. What about the chin-up bar you bought one night while watching the infomercial on TV? I know, by the time it came in the mail you had lost interest or you just didn't have time to assemble it (a five-minute job) and start benefiting from its use. You must have a stack of books you can get your hands on, perfect for hopping over, back and forth, in beat to your favorite music.

Speaking of good music, why don't you try turning on some tunes and dance next time you're doing housework? It goes a lot faster that way and it's loads of fun! Just turn the music up and dance! You'll be working out for an hour (more or less depending on the size of your house and how obsessive you are), but it'll feel like you're dancing at a party! Play some upbeat music, like salsa, merengue, hip-hop, oldies, or whatever makes your feet start tapping. Then just start shaking it! Once you get going, you may just keep going until the entire house is clean as a whistle.

While you take a break and are on the phone or watching TV, work those calves. Lift up and down on your calves 20 times with your feet facing forward, then do 20 more with your feet facing outward, and 20 more with your feet facing inward. Build those muscles! And you've never left the house.

In fact, when's the last time you used that bike in your garage? If you don't have a bike, you can probably find a used one pretty cheap online. So no excuses there.

If you're thinking about lifting weights, no need to join a gym, especially when money is tight. While there's no doubt that a fitness center provides many benefits, most of the exercise you really need can be accomplished in your home and in your neighborhood.

Determining your goals (and your family's) is essential to creating a fun fitness plan that is reasonable and maintainable. Is it weight loss you're after? Are you genetically predisposed to an illness or condition that exercise and weight loss would prevent (or at least make the condition more manageable)? Do you want to gain definition and muscle mass or merely tone up? Are you hoping to sleep better and avoid chronic digestive issues? Whatever your reasons for exercising, what's most important is consistent effort and flexible programming. Make movement of

The Family Training Zone

any kind a habit, but be creative with what activities you choose to include in your daily diet.

When's the last time you put on some of your favorite music, cleared a little space, and just had fun dancing? There are so many opportunities for you right in your home to improve your overall condition.

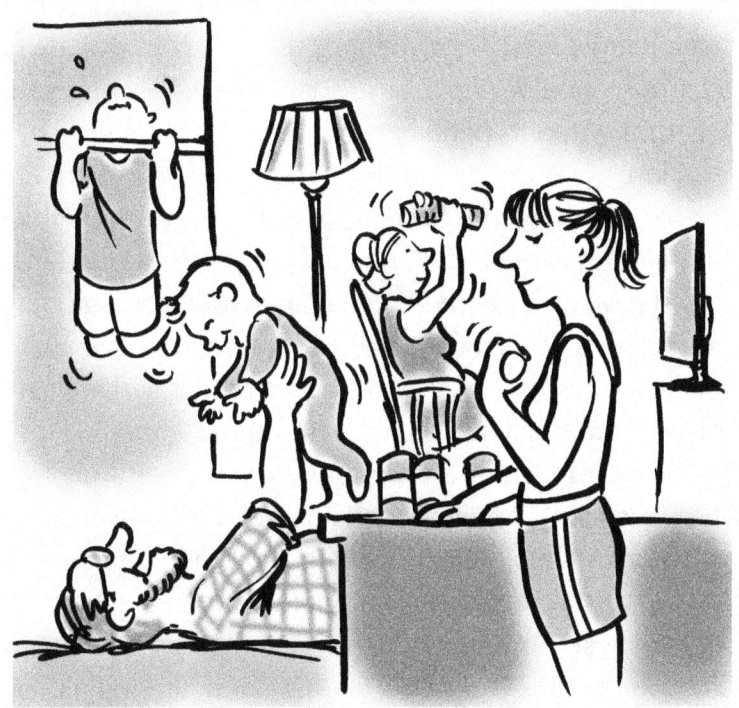

There's a hidden gym inside everyone's house. You'd be surprised how easy it can be to get in shape right there under your own roof.

Pass the Paint Can and Other Family Games

Whether you own a house, rent an apartment, or share space in a mobile home, everyone has done some painting at one time or another in his or her residence. Invariably, you're stuck with leftover paint, often by the gallon. If you wrap an old washcloth around the metal handle to protect your hands, you've got weights to lift. If the paint can is nearly empty, fill it with water or dirt and you're ready to go. Curls, shoulder rolls, arm extensions—all are at your fingertips without spending a penny.

Here's a game to play with your family. Take a paint can, small or large, depending on the age and strength of your kids, and see how long you can pass it around in a circle before you get tired. Remember your starting point, by time or by revolutions, and see how you can eventually build on your record. As you all get stronger and improve your endurance, you can increase the weight.

What about those stairs in your house or building? There are plenty of games and competitions you can create, using a simple flight of stairs. How many times can you go up and down in one minute? How many times in five minutes? How long does it take to hop up and down? On one leg? The variety is endless, and as long as you are moving and having fun (and probably working up a good sweat) then it's well worth the effort.

> **Thank You**
>
> To Sarah Stokes, a certified ZUMBA® instructor, living and working in Houston, for her helpful tips and ideas, woven into this chapter.

Family Boot Camp

While some families prefer this random, playful approach, others may prefer a more disciplined, programmed system of exercise. Welcome to boot camp, family style.

Basic training in the military begins with a morning run. It may be too much to ask most families to get up in unison and run five miles, especially right off the bat, but what's keeping all of you from getting up ten minutes earlier than usual and running around the block a few times? Ten minutes earlier out of bed can translate so easily into ten minutes of jogging around the neighborhood or a chunk of push-ups, sit-ups, and jumping jacks. The benefits of these good, old-fashioned exercises are obvious. The trick is to do them on a regular basis. If you can accomplish that, the joy of doing them together as a family is yours to discover.

Once you and your family get active in your own backyard, why not extend the fun to your local park, discovering what's there that's fun, and challenging—individually and as a family. To spice things up, visit your high school running track and see how you can take running, jogging, or speed-walking, to another level.

The Wright Choice

If you're a parent of a teenager, you may be wondering how you can get your kid to put down her cell phone long enough to stop texting and get fit. It might feel like a losing battle and while we don't condone texting and running (or walking, for that matter) at the same time, you may try cajoling your child into handing over their portable "it's my world and welcome to it" device and seeing how many laps they can run around an oval track without stopping to check their phone.

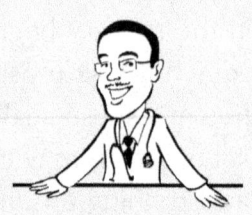

RANDY'S RULES
Pick Your Battles.
No matter what situation you are in with your kids, you must determine what's worth fighting about and what's better to simply let go, at least for another day.

The Dining Room Table Workout

Take your normal 6 p.m. dinnertime and push it back to 6:15, or better still, 6:30. That leaves 15 to 30 minutes for family exercise, ensuring some excellent appetites. Everybody has been sitting most of the day—in school, at the office, in the car, or wherever—and you all need to get up and move before sitting even more during the evening.

The Family Training Zone

The five exercises here take about five minutes to complete so they can be done easily, together as a family, right there at your dining room table, just before you eat. No excuses. No special equipment. Just follow the illustrations and simple instructions.

1. Table Push-up (only for those with solid, secure tables that won't slide or break)

Focus: Upper Body, Shoulders, Arms, and Chest

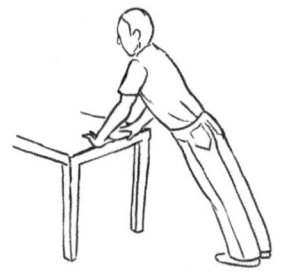 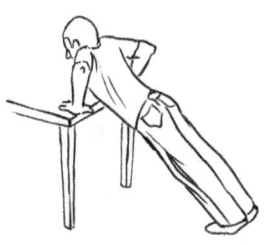

Keep your hands shoulder-width apart and your body straight. Slowly lower your chest to the table and return to the starting position.
Repeat.
Start with three, progress to five, and try seven by the end of the week.

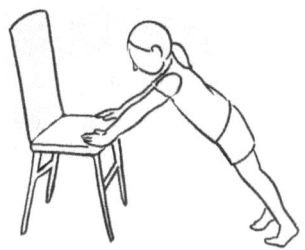 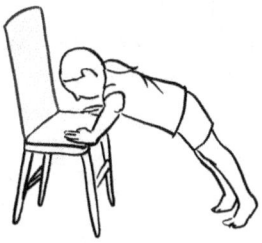

Children can do the same thing, using a chair securely placed so it won't slide.

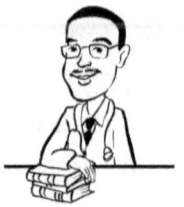

THE WRIGHT ADVICE
Adjust the degree of difficulty according to age, size, and capability.
Everyone should be comfortable but challenged.

2. Back Extension
Focus: Core Muscles, Abs, Thighs, and Hips

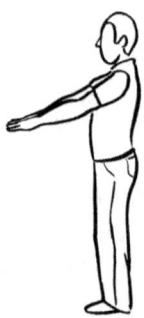 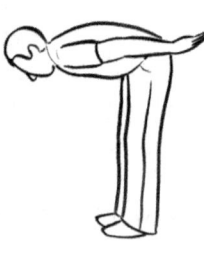

Stand with your feet shoulder-width apart. Keep your back straight as you slowly bend over to a 90-degree position. Return slowly to your starting posture. Start with five repetitions and work your way up to ten. You may even try to touch your toes!

The Family Training Zone

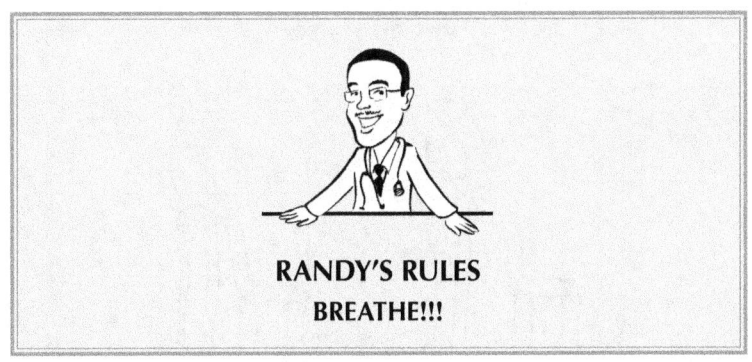

RANDY'S RULES
BREATHE!!!

3. Table Squat
Focus: Lower Body, Legs, Hips, and Calves

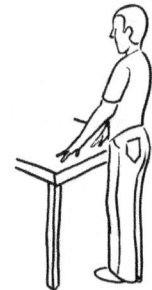 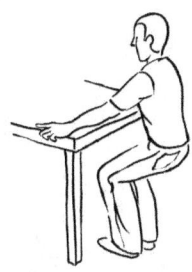

Stand in front of a table, with your feet parallel. Bend your knees as pictured, with your arms extended straight ahead for balance. Start with five and work your way up to ten.

4. Calf Raise

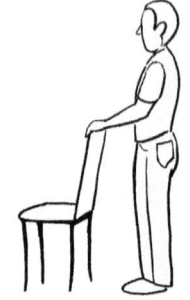 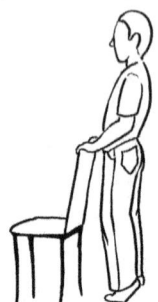

*Stand with your feet together, holding on to the back of a chair. Raise up on both feet, as if trying to stand on your toes. To make it harder, try one leg at a time.
Begin with five and progress to ten.*

5. Chair Twist
Focus: Stretching, Flexibility, Stress Relief

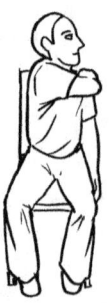 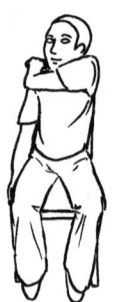

While sitting straight in your chair, with your feet flat on the floor, place your left hand on the front corner of the seat of your chair. Extend your right arm straight out at shoulder level and across your chest. Place your right hand on the opposite back seat rest of your chair. Keep your head still and look straight ahead. Hold this position for ten seconds and release. Repeat this sequence with the opposite hand.

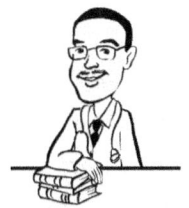

THE WRIGHT ADVICE
Whenever possible, add your own ideas to these exercises.
You may have seen an exercise video,
or your children may have learned something in school.

"Exergamming"

It's no secret that parents can grow desperate on a rainy weekend day, trying to keep their kids entertained. Even in an age of overwhelming technology, kids can't spend the entire day in front of a computer or the family TV. Or can they? Many teenagers are capable of staying on Facebook for hours at a time. Younger kids can, too. So, if most children are almost uncontrollably attracted to whatever they can find on their computers or TVs, why not offer them something really beneficial?

There is a growing body of research supporting "exergamming" as a viable way to increase activity for children who lead a sedentary life. It's not a substitute for good old-fashioned sports, like jogging, playing basketball or tennis, but it sure is better than sitting on the couch for hours, shooting space aliens like I used to do in high school!

Exergamming is a way to engage your child's desire to play while helping him to move, move, move! Why not surprise your media-savvy kids the next time you are at the store and offer to buy them a video game? Buy one that is very active, incorporating dancing, running, and jumping! If you play with them on a regular basis (if they let you!), this would be a great way to be "hip" in their eyes, spend some quality time with them, and burn a few calories in the process!

Yoga

If traditional exercise, such as weightlifting, jogging, and recreational athletics is not for you, then why not try yoga? For centuries, yoga has been a valuable centerpiece for healthy living, both in a physical and spiritual sense. More and more people around the country are getting on board, signing up for yoga classes at their local gyms and attending centers devoted entirely to its practice.

Ask your kids. Some of them are participating in yoga classes at school, both during the day as part of the core curriculum and in after-school programs. Take a moment to observe your children in a yoga program, and you'll probably be inspired to join them.

But some of you may be wondering, what is yoga, exactly?

Yoga refers to a traditional physical and mental discipline originating in India. The Sanskrit word "yoga" has many meanings and is derived from the Sanskrit root yuj, meaning "to control," "to yoke," or "to unite." Outside India, the term yoga is typically associated with hatha yoga and its asanas (postures) as a form of exercise. It is a healing system of theory and practice, which has been around more than five thousand years. It combines breathing exercises, physical postures and meditation. Western forms of yoga typically focus more on the physical aspects. The more rigorous styles of yoga practiced in the United States are referred to as ashtanga and power yoga, which involve a constant flow of postures designed to challenge your body and provide a total body workout. Generally, the more traditional yogi will practice hatha style, which involves a set pattern of specific asanas, which are held for a set period of time combined with the breath.

The benefits of yoga include increased flexibility, muscle strengthening, better posture, body awareness, and the ability to focus. Yoga is an ageless form of exercise that allows babies, children, adults, and elderly to work out at any stage of life. Information and classes are readily available at most gyms and yoga centers or can be practiced at home through books, and videos, or by viewing exercise programs on television.

> A special thanks to Roslyn Brazzelle,
> yoga instructor and founder of PIYOLET,
> for her generous contribution to this section.

What Is PIYOLET?

PIYOLET is PI-Pilates, YO-Yoga, and LET-Ballet, fused together to create a low-impact, fun, and invigorating workout for the entire body. PIYOLET allows you to reshape and redefine your appearance while encouraging a positive and healthy lifestyle. Each of the disciplines has numerous benefits.

Pilates, the physical fitness system developed in the early twentieth century by Joseph Pilates, focuses on the core postural muscles with the goal of strengthening the deep torso muscles, maintaining a balanced body, and providing support for the spine. We've discussed yoga. Ballet has been practiced for centuries and traditionally involves the discipline, balance, and flow of precise acrobatic and dance movements, with the accompaniment of classical music.

The benefits of PIYOLET include weight loss, muscle strengthening, increased flexibility, improved balance, lengthening of the muscles, better posture, and core toning, all while relaxing and refreshing the mind, body, and spirit.

No tutus, ballet shoes, or special equipment necessary.

Meditation

When many of us hear the word "meditation," we may conjure up images of Buddhist monks performing a strict and sober discipline in some remote retreat away from what we call civilization. While there are plenty of spiritually inclined people devoted to meditation as part of their religious practice, more and more regular folks are learning about the physical, emotional, and psychological benefits that meditation—even a small amount—can provide. In fact, some of them may even be practicing meditation right in your neighborhood—behind closed doors or in the backyard on a nice day. While most people associate running, swimming, biking, sports, and exercise (weights, aerobics, etc.) with getting (and staying) fit, meditation is often overlooked for its purely physical attributes. Don't underestimate the value of stillness, control, and proper breathing.

These principles, so integral to yoga, are also the starting points for learning meditation. Just a few minutes a day can make a remarkable difference in your overall well-being.

Now, let's learn more about this ancient ritual and how it can make sense in our everyday lives.

Meditation is a process of focusing on one thing at a time. It's like trying to get good reception on your television, only this time it's you you're tuning. Meditation trains your body, mind, and emotions to work together. When this occurs, the more in tune you become, and the static, interference, and fuzziness in your life will begin to disappear. You will find that you have more energy and feel happier.

To assist this process, check your state of being before and after each practice. Without changing anything, just close your eyes. Begin to observe how you are in this moment.

This kind of play is our first meditation, and happiness just arises, not from what we are doing, but from how we are. As our idle thoughts cease, peace and well-being enter. Whenever we devote ourselves fully to something or someone, we are already meditating. Activities that take a degree of concentration, like golf and needlepoint, are popular because they remind us of this state. No matter what the activity is, it is the quality of our connection to it that is important. Meditation develops this ability to connect deeply with anything or anyone.

The calm, happy state of heightened awareness that comes in meditating is actually the natural state of your being. Children experience this state spontaneously. Just watch how a child focuses on something he or she loves.

> **THANKS**
> To Rory Pinto,
> a spiritual healer and meditation specialist from New York City and the founder of *Inner Resources*, for his contribution to this section.

Thoughts to Ponder and Practice

Before you can change any condition, you first have to become aware of it. As you tune in to your comfort level, you will know the degree of change that you can handle, and you will not proceed too far or too fast. Like eating in a balanced way, you can take in only so much at one time, and you have to allow time to digest and assimilate before you can take in any more. Notice how you speed up or slow down the process of change.

A key to facilitating this lies in allowing change to happen in its own way, at its own pace, rather than forcing the method and speed. You lead by following, making moment-to-moment corrections to your course by staying aware, by literally staying in touch. As soon as any forcing enters the process, a conflict is created and your body becomes tense. Your job is just to keep watching your own process of unfolding and love yourself in whatever state you find yourself!

A Mini-Meditation
(For Busy People on the Go Who Need to Slow Down)

Begin by really feeling your feet on the floor. As you continue to feel your feet, include another sensation: the feeling of clothes on your skin. Realize the feeling of the air playing on your hands and face.

Now, include the feeling of the weight of your body on the chair. Watch the rising and falling of your breath, without having to fix or change anything. Notice whether it is long or short, deep or shallow, smooth or ragged.

Using your sense of touch, feel your body as a whole. Feel it all at once. Feel your body having weight, taking up space, having density, and all these sensations.

While still feeling your body with all its sensations, let the listening run out and let it hold all of the sounds in the environment for a while, near and far, not clinging to any one sound, not pushing any sound away.

This mini-meditation (one to three minutes) is best done before and after an activity. It helps you to focus before you begin, and regroup after you have completed it. When practiced throughout the day this pause will refresh you and prevent the build-up of tension and fatigue. By bringing your awareness out of your thoughts and into your body, the practice helps to integrate your mental state with your physical state. The calmness and strength that arise allow ease, poise, and efficiency to come into your work and play.

The Mindfulness of Breathing
(For Families Who Eat Too Fast and Can't Get to Sleep!)

The mindfulness of breathing is a basic concentration practice. It brings rest to your mind and body. When the mind wanders or is distracted, bring your focus back to the sensations that you experience as you breathe.

Don't try to control the breath. Just watch it. Slow or fast, deep or shallow; what matters is not the quality of the breath, but the quality of your attention.

When you are comfortable, begin to scan your body, and become aware of any physical sensations you may encounter. Go to one sensation at a time, feel it, and take it in. Stay neutral: neither clinging to it nor pushing it away.

Work down your body with awareness and continue to watch and experience each sensation. Let it go and move on to the next one.

Once you have scanned the entire body, begin at the head and be aware of any sensations that you may encounter. Include any emotions that you may come upon.

Focus on one sensation at a time. Give it a name if you wish and move on to the next one. As you become aware of each sensation, feeling, or thought, bring love and kindness to it.

A Standing Meditation
(For Busy Families on the Go Who Need to Calm Down!)

Stand relaxed, with your knees slightly bent, legs shoulder-width apart, and hands at your sides. Allow your fingers to gently curve and remain slightly apart. Drop your shoulders and let your arms hang loosely. Relax your hips and belly. Your weight should be evenly balanced between front and rear, and from side to side. Your tailbone is tipped slightly forward. Your tongue is touching the roof of your mouth, behind your teeth. Your eyes are looking forward and slightly down.

Imagine a line coming from the sky attached to a point in the top center of your head (on line with the tips of the ears), keeping your posture erect and balanced, without being rigid or floppy. Imagine this line continuing down the center of your body and connecting to a round sphere of light a little larger than a golf ball. This sphere is at a level of two inches below your navel, sitting right in front of the spinal column. This is a reservoir for your subtle energy, called the Tantien.

Imagine that, like a puppet, your whole body is suspended from your head. Feel yourself sinking down, relaxing, as you hang from the string. Breathe calmly and naturally. Exhale completely and allow your chest to drop. Let the feeling of standing in this relaxed, alert way sink in.

Stand quietly, for up to five minutes.

As simple as this practice appears, it will quickly expose your level of nervous tension, how high-strung you are, and any difficulty you may have in relaxing. It is very humbling. You will find that as you practice, your nervous system will settle down and become more calm, laying a foundation for a deeper connection with yourself and a better relationship with others, in your family and in your community at large.

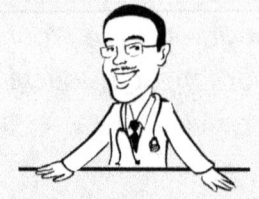

RANDY'S RULES

STOP SMOKING!

If you smoke inside your house,
where your spouse and children live,
turn yourself in immediately!

No joke.

You need help.

You all do.

Stop hurting innocent people,
especially your own family.

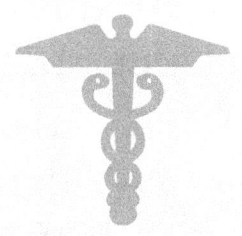

The Wright Reminders

Get 30 minutes of exercise every day.

Breathe!

Do not smoke.

Engage your family in an exercise program.

Enjoy your body!

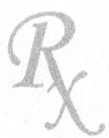

STOP!

EXERCISE BREAK!

You were probably so busy reading about exercise that you didn't actually do any while reading this chapter.

It's never too late.

And not very hard, unless you made it that way, which is also recommended if you can handle it.

Especially when it's only a minimum of 25 little minutes.

Ah, go ahead, make it 30.

That way, when you get to the next (and last) chapter, you won't be surprised.

CHAPTER **15**

Home Sweet Home

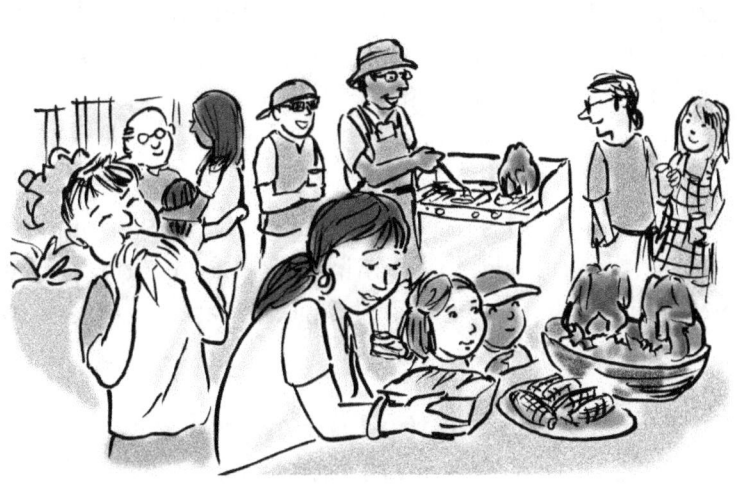

Medical Myth #10
"It'll never happen to me!"

It? You mean a stroke, a heart attack, or a sudden diagnosis of diabetes? Based upon all my years as a doctor, and without even having met you, not knowing your age, history, or physical condition, I can say with all certainty that yes—it can happen to you. And if it's not you, it can unfortunately be someone you love who becomes afflicted by any number of ailments and/or life-threatening situations. All myths aside, it can happen to anyone—at anytime.

So what does one do? We have faith in ourselves that we will do the right thing, meaning eating right and getting fit. For many of us, we have faith in some higher power that looks after us in one fashion or another. We pray. We celebrate our life each day and, hopefully, we fill our time with joy and love.

Armed with a better sense of your goals, the knowledge of what food is really made of, and an understanding of the risks you take by ignoring this information, you're probably ready to embrace change. What better place to start than in your own home?

Welcome the Portion Police to Your Dinner Table

The family that eats together often eats too much! We've already announced that the first rule of healthy eating is to know how much you are ingesting! But in all honesty, one look around and it's clear that this instruction bears repeating. For the casual shopper, serving size can be the first trap that leads to excessive eating.

The information on the nutritional label is based on one serving size. If you are drinking a 12-ounce soda, and the listed serving size is 6 ounces, it means that there are two servings in the bottle or can and you have to double all the values to get an accurate picture of what you are putting into your body. In other words, if the soda lists 60 calories per serving, and you drink the whole container, then you're actually drinking 120 calories! This can sometimes be tricky (I dare not say deceptive), because most people assume that when they see the number of calories per serving, this means for the whole bottle (or package) and fail to look at the serving size.

The cardinal rule is read carefully and always size up your food!

The New American Plate

Congratulations. You have learned about the nature, risks, and benefits of the various nutrients you eat. Now, let's start developing a specific meal plan for you and your family. With that in mind, I would like to ask you to keep an open mind about a new way to think about eating.

Americans traditionally view meat as the cornerstone of our dinner plate (or even lunch) and consider veggies a side dish. On top of that, as our country continues to embrace the idea of "bigger means better" our concept of an appropriate portion size has increased to seriously unhealthy proportions. Unfortunately, our appetites seem to have grown exponentially. We simply want more and more food. In a society that is also obsessed with convenience, it is easy to see why obesity has become such an epidemic. We move less and eat more, which is a perfect recipe for disaster.

The insidious part is that these habits develop slowly so we often don't notice them until it's too late. In fact, many people notice symptoms of bad health but they choose to ignore those developments. As a society, we seem to have done just that.

Luckily, the American Institute for Cancer Research (AICR) has recognized these negative trends in our collective behavior and reacted with a remarkably simple approach to decreasing our risk for cancer, heart disease, and stroke (to mention but a few life-threatening conditions), as well as improving our overall health.

It's simple common sense based on science. No one is preaching about going to the ends of the earth to find that one rare plant to cure all our ills; it's a simple eating plan that anyone can begin immediately.

The AICR's New American Plate suggests that we make meat a side dish and use fruit and veggies as our main staples. Officially, it calls for our plates to consist mainly of vegetables, fruit, whole grains, and beans. This may be a difficult concept for many of my fellow Texans to imagine, since beef is king here. That's why, like everything in this book, change should be made slowly. The AICR suggests transitioning slowly until meat occupies only one third of your plate at any given meal.

You can visit its website at www.aicr.org.

> **STOP!**
> **EXERCISE BREAK!**
>
> While you're trying to come up with that list, it's time for your exercise break.
> That'll burn off some of the fat you've eaten so far today.
> 30 minutes—minimum.
> You made it. You've reached the target of 30 minutes of exercise each and every day.
> KEEP IT UP!

Raising Food-Responsible Children

There is a lot of money and political effort going toward changing how schools deal with the health of our children. With the rates of childhood obesity on a relentless rise, something must be done to literally save our children. I suggest that we start at home, long before our children even enter the hallways of their school!

Chef Bobo, who runs the kitchen at The Calhoun School in New York City, says "parents can be a powerful force in supporting kids' healthy eating by not having processed foods available at home. Snacks should be nuts, fruits, granola, popcorn, etc. Healthy eating can also be supported by eating family meals together a couple times a week, preferably prepared as a joint effort by all members of the family."

It is our obligation as parents to raise our children to be as healthy as possible, and that includes learning to be physically active and making the right choices about food. So why is it so difficult? As our kids grow up, we teach them the basics about financial responsibility, so why can't we do a better job of teaching them the nuts and bolts of *gastronomic* responsibility? We should be instructing our children to handle their plates with just as much care as we handle our checkbooks! We must guide them toward understanding the psychology of food and becoming responsible for what they eat, how much, and when.

That would be true *gastronomic* responsibility.

When Saying Grace Means Slowing Down

When I say grace, by myself, at home with my family, or at the office with my staff and visitors who may be joining us for lunch, it's my way of giving thanks to God for providing me with a meal to enjoy and the company to enjoy it with.

You would be surprised by the reactions I get when I take a moment to pray in public before a meal. I never thought of it until I prayed at the office with some visitors, many of them from various religious backgrounds and beliefs.

My prayers consist mainly of giving thanks for the life of myself, my family, and my friends. In that moment, all of the day's craziness slows down and we are still, giving us the chance to be mindful of the food we are about to eat and how it arrived on our plates. For me, it is a meditative action, which I am quite sure contributes to my continued good health, both physically and spiritually.

I am not suggesting that saying grace is appropriate for everyone. But I would ask you, as I do all my patients when searching for a complete diagnosis, to examine your life and see if a moment of grace may be a missing factor in your ultra-busy world. And looking honestly at your situation at home, are you really one big, happy family? If so, great! But if not, if your family is not operating so well together, how can you identify the issues and acquire the necessary tools to affect positive, long-lasting changes? How can you come to create these moments of grace in your house?

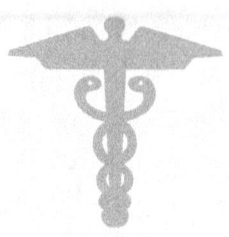

The Wright Reminders

Enlist the portion police at home.

Eat meat as a side dish.

Slow down at the family dinner table.

Commit to good health.

No more excuses!

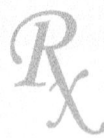

Conclusion
A Call to Action

A Beautiful Transformation

Putting this book together has been an inspirational journey. I have met some amazing people along the way, and as I have learned more and more about living a healthier lifestyle I have grown even more committed to sharing that message with others. Above all, I have come to realize one essential thing.

Despite our society's obsession with "personal growth," we are a family, whether it's at home, within our community, at a church, in a city, or even a nation. Each of us is part of something greater than ourselves. Despite our perceived differences, we are linked by a common lineage and humanity, and for that reason your health does matter to me, just as mine should matter to you! The healthier your family is at home, the healthier you will be. The healthier your community is, the healthier you will also be! It is your responsibility not only to help yourselves and your family become healthier, but you must help your community become healthier as well!

How do you do that? It starts with simple communication. Discuss what you have learned in this book with your friends, coworkers, and church members. Start a conversation with someone standing in line at the store. Be curious. Lead by example! Just like praying in public may call attention to your actions, eating healthy food in public will often do the same. Taking a moment to stretch might do observers as much of a favor as you're doing yourself. People are watching you! Why not inspire them?

Conclusion: A Call to Action

When someone asks about what you are doing or eating, use that moment to share some life-saving tips. You never know who you'll be helping or how important one little comment may be.

If you use social media, like Facebook or YouTube, post pictures of the new recipes you just prepared and share the comments you receive about the benefits your choices have to offer. It's great to "fix" yourself and your family, but why not share all that you're learning with others? You'll be happy to discover that there are many people out there looking to be inspired, and once you get the ball rolling, the rewards will reveal themselves as they come back to you.

How's Your Reading Comprehension?

This is a test. Of course it is. Why would we try to teach you all this stuff if we didn't want you to remember as much of it as possible?

Remember that litmus test in Chapter 1? Let's see how you do now, after reading this book, doing further research on your own, and seeing your doctor.

1. How many people in my family have a history of heart disease?

2. What is my normal weight, blood pressure, and cholesterol count?

3. What weighs more, muscle or fat?

4. What's in a fastfood burger?

Conclusion: A Call to Action

5. How many children in America are obese?

6. What's a carbohydrate?

7. Where does protein come from, and what does it do?

8. What is trans fat?

9. How many calories should I eat, on average, each day?

10. What is in a multivitamin?

Goals, Goals, Goals

How's your To Do list coming along? Remember those long-term goals you wrote down at the end of Chapter 1? Considering all that we hope you have learned reading this book, please use this space to revise your goals, if necessary.

Creating a Health Contract for You and Your Family

It's your job to take control of your life. It's your job, as a parent, to guide your children toward doing the same thing as they get older and leave the nest. Wishing for things to be different will not change anything. Complaining will not either.

Change is your responsibility. Stop waiting for someone else to fix health care. True and lasting health care reform starts in your mind! Every time you make a healthy choice or help someone else do the same, you are saving our nation money by reducing the risk of disease. As you change, so will others, and you can keep each other accountable for maintaining your improvements. It is more fun to do things in groups, so the more public you make your changes and the more people you draw in, the easier it will be to sustain your changes! In essence, you must become the change! Each of us, in this respect, can be a leader, starting in our own house and extending out into our communities.

Conclusion: A Call to Action

When we marry, we sign a contract, agreeing to love, honor, and respect our partner. It feels effortless when we feel we have met the right person. When we begin a new job, we often sign a contract, pledging our best professional integrity, honesty, and commitment. When our children go to school, they promise to behave in the classroom and do their best to promote cooperation, good sportsmanship, and hard work. All three of these contracts potentially bind us to a greater place in life and raise the bar for a higher quality of living. Isn't it time you created a health contract for yourself and your family where you openly commit to living a healthier, wealthier, and wiser life? It's your choice, and now is your time to make the most of it.

Good luck and good health. You're in charge of at least one of them.

The Wright Choice

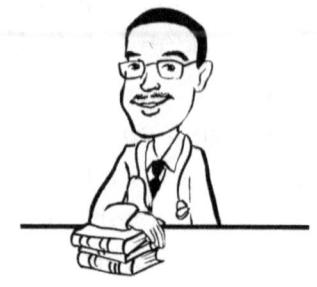

DR. WRIGHT'S PRESCRIPTION FOR BUSY FAMILIES ON THE GO

1. Examine your lifestyle. This is your first step toward getting healthy.

2. Create a family Bill of Health that you can practice daily.

3. Learn about the foods you eat and raise "health smart" children.

4. Be a heart healthy shopper and learn to read labels. EYE it b4 U buy it!

5. Throw Away Yours Scales! It's not how much you lose—it's how you lose it.

Conclusion: A Call to Action

6. Find the hidden gym in your house and make exercise a family affair.

7. Remodel your environment— at home, at work, and at play.

8. Be open-minded. Explore new foods and fitness fun.

9. Be patient. Make each choice the right choice.

10. Inspire your community and help the world get healthy.

Index

adenosine, 113
adult-onset diabetes. *See* type 2 diabetes.
aerobic conditioning, 380
after-school snacks, healthy, 346–7
alcohol
    heart disease and, 100
    moderation with, 348
    sleep and, 116
American Academy of Pediatrics recommendations, 170
American Dietary Association recommendations, 195
American Heart Association recommendations, 55, 154, 166–8, 186–7, 189, 195, 244, 266–70
American Institute for Cancer Research recommendations, 107, 408
amino acids
    energy from, 145
    protein and, 144–5, 147
    supplements, 155
antibiotics, in food, 247–8, 250
Arceneaux, Chester, 11
artificial sweeteners, 365
at-home exercise, 383–6
atherosclerosis. *See* heart disease.

back extensions, 390
bakery departments, grocery stores', 243–4
Banschick, Mark, 10, 110, 175–6
beer, non-alcoholic, 362
beverages
    alcoholic, 100, 116, 348
    healthy, 216–7
    non-alcoholic, 352
    sugary, 268
Big Mac, nutritional content of, 75
Blackman, Patrick, 276
blenders, 289
BLTs, 309–11
    Not Your Mama's BLT, 301
Body Mass Index, 54–5
body test, 376
bottled water, quality of, 212–4
brain, strokes and, 98–9
bran, grain, 135–6, 138
Brazzelle, Roslyn, 395
breads
    healthy, 134–6, 244
    white, 136–9, 244
    whole grain, 134–5, 244
breakfast
    energy depleting vs. boosting, 129
    recipes, 280–290

breathing, mindfulness of, 400–1
brown rice, nutritional content of, 139
brunch recipes, 292–300
budgeting, healthy eating and, 260, 264–5
butter, choosing, 246
Butterfield, Gail, 150

caffeine, sleep and, 113–15
calf raises, 392
calories
    burned during exercise, 380–1
    burned in daily activities, 186–9
    counting, 189, 230–1
    daily requirements for, 184–5, 187
    defined, 182–3
    discretionary, 189–90
    excess stored as fat, 183. *See also* under glucose.
    liquid, 191
    solid, 191
cancer
    basics of, 104–8
    diet and, 139
    prevention of, 107–8, 139
carbohydrates
    complex, 124–9, 133–4
    daily value of, 228
    glucose derived from, 129–30
    health benefits of, 139–40
    "low carb" diets and, 123, 131–3, 138–9, 150
    misperceptions about, 123–4
    Recommended Dietary Allowance of, 133
    refined, 136
    simple, 124–5
    sources of good, 133–4, 140
chair twists, 392
children
    after-school snacks for, 346–7
    aversion to vegetables, 299
    childhood obesity, combating, 87–91
    encouraging health habits in, 175–7, 306–7, 409–10
    exercise and, 377–9, 387–8
    milk consumption and, 170, 246, 307–8
    nutrition for, 307–8, 312, 314
    peer pressure and, 177
    psychological complexes and, 110–11
    role modeling health habits for, 175–7
    school lunches and, 302–3, 306–7
charcoal grills, 359
"chiptons," 327
cholesterol
    chemistry of, 170
    heart disease and, 170, 172–4
    LDL, 163, 172–8
    meat and, 270
    ranges, 171
communities, building health habits in, 414–5
complex carbohydrates
    chemistry of, 124–5
    diet high in, 129
    nutritional value of, 126–8
    sources of, 133–4
conditioning, breaking, 7–9
Confucius, 27
cooking oils, healthy, 246, 319
cooking sprays, 287
Cordua, David, 276, 313

Index

Cosgrove, Delos M., 92
crackers, healthy, 328
crepes, 283–5
   Crepe Ambrosia with Sauce Ala Orange, 283
culture, health habits and, 36–7, 71–2

dairy
   protein from, 148
   section of grocery store, 245–6
Daniel (prophet), 81
dehydration, 145, 150
denial
   childhood complexes and, 110–11
   health consequences of, 14–16, 86–7
desserts, 364
diabetes
   basics of, 101–4
   diet and, 104, 126
   exercise and, 104
   glucose and, 102–4, 125
   high Glycemic-Index foods and, 126
   obesity and, 104
   type-1, 102–3
   type-2, 88, 103, 139
diets
   lacto-ovo vegetarian, 153
   "low carb," 123, 131–3, 138–9, 150
   macrobiotic, 146
   vegan, 149, 153, 195, 329
   vegetarian, 149, 153, 176–7, 195
   For dieting, see weight loss.
Dietary Reference Intake, 133
dinner recipes, 332–41
discretionary calories, 189–90

dog walking, 377
doggy bags, restaurant, 259–60
Dubner, Anne, 78–9, 128, 239, 265–6, 276–7, 310

Economic Research Service, USDA's, 250
egg yolks, using, 328
Einstein, Albert, 90
endosperm, grain, 135–6, 138
Environmental Protection Agency, 211–12
Environmental Working Group report, 210–11
exercise
   at-home, 383–92
   body tests and, 376
   calories burned during, 380–1
   children and, 377–9, 387–8, 393–4
   "exergamming and," 393–4
   family, 387–8
   heart rate during, 381–3
   muscle-strengthening, 376–7
   Pilates and, 396
   PIYOLET and, 396
   recommendations for daily, 374, 379
   tips for, 379–80
   yoga as, 394–5
"exergamming," 393–4

Family Food Diary, 62–4
family medical histories, importance of, 32–9
fast food
   habitual consumption of, 69, 73
   health costs of, 258–9
   nutritional content of, 74, 76, 78–9, 85

425

fats
  amino acids and, 145
  appeal of fatty foods and, 160–2
  daily intake of, 78–9
  excess energy storage and, 125, 126–7, 130–1, 183
  food labels and, 231
  healthy, 162–3, 285, 319
  milk and, 169
  monounsaturated fats and, 162–3, 319
  nuts and, 285
  omega-3, 154, 163, 244, 251, 267, 285
  omega-6, 163
  polyunsaturated fats, 162–3
  saturated fats and, 168–9, 228, 269–70
  trans fats and, 165–8, 248
fat loss, science behind, 132–3
fertilizers, in food, 249–50
fiber
  daily value of, 228
  nutritional value of, 126–8
  sources of, 134
filtration systems, water, 214–5
fish
  omega-3 fatty acids and, 154, 244, 267, 285
  protein from, 154
  servings per week, 267
flexibility training, 380
food allergies, dining out and, 255
Food and Farm Act, 251
food labels
  calorie counts and, 230–1
  Daily Value and, 226–8
  fat content and, 231
  importance of, 224–5
  interpreting, 226–8
  percent of Daily Value and, 226, 228
  serving sizes and, 229–30, 407
food pyramid, USDA's, 184–5, 314
fructose, 124
fruits
  cancer prevention and, 107–8
  getting children to eat, 306–7
  shopping for, 243
  servings per day, 267
  source of carbohydrates, 133–4
  source of fiber, 127

galactose, 124
gas grills, 359
Genealogical Health Charts, 38–9
genetics, role of, 32, 36. *See also* family medical histories.
germ, grain, 135–6, 138
gestational diabetes, basics of, 103–4
glucose
  amino acids and, 145
  carbohydrates and, 129–30
  chemistry of, 124
  diabetes and, 102–4, 125
  excess stored as fat, 125, 126, 130
  protein and, 130
  soluble fibers and, 128
goals, health
  defining, 26–8
  setting, 21, 418
God's view of us, 11
Glycemic Index
  foods high on, 125–6
  soluble fiber and, 128

Index

glycogen
　excess glucose storage and, 126–7, 130
　lost through low carb diets, 132
grace, before meals, 410–11
grass-fed animals, 250–1
grilling, 358–63
　choosing a grill and, 359
　recipes for, 360–3
grills, charcoal vs. gas, 359
Grocery Manufacturers Association, advertising of, 73
grocery shopping
　plan for, 241–6
　shopping lists and, 234, 242

HDL cholesterol, lowered atherosclerosis risk and, 172–4
health contract, family's, 418–9
heart disease
　alcohol consumption and, 100
　basics of, 100–1
　cholesterol and, 170, 172–4
　diet and, 139
　monounsaturated fats and, 163
　prevalence of, 374
　preventing, 100–1, 139, 172–4
　smoking and, 100
heart rate, calculating, 381–3
Holley, Mark, 254–5, 265, 276, 309–10, 322, 358
honey, as sugar substitute, 365
"Hoppin John," 322
hormones, in food, 247–8, 250
hot dogs, nutritional content of, 76, 78–9
household products, healthy, 247
husks, grain, 135–6

hydrogenated fats, 166. See also trans fats.

insoluble fibers, 128
insomnia, 114
insulin
　high Glycemic-Index foods and, 125–6
　role in diabetes, 102–3, 125
insulin resistance, high Glycemic Index foods and, 126

julienning, 335
junk food, nutritional content of, 73–9
juvenile diabetes. See type 1 diabetes.

Laborers' Health and Safety Fund of North America, 188
lacto-ovo vegetarian diet, 153. See also vegetarian diet.
LDL cholesterol
　atherosclerosis risk and, 172–4
　monounsaturated fats and, 163
learned helplessness, 7–9
leftovers
　good use of, 271–2, 300, 364
　safety of, 343–4
legumes, servings per week, 269
Life Style Assessment, 18–19
likes and dislikes, personal, 24–6
liquid calories, 191
locally grown food, 250–1
"low carb" diets, 123, 131–3, 138–9, 150
lunch
　recipes for, 306–15, 318–22, 324–30
　school lunches and, 302–3, 306–7

427

lunchmeat, 234, 245

macaroni and cheese, healthy vs. unhealthy, 342–3
macrobiotic diets, 149
margarines, trans fats in, 246
mason jars, 359
meal planning
    incorporating leftovers into, 271–2, 300, 364
    menus, 368–70
    new eating habits and, 407–8
    recipes. See separate entry.
    taste vs. health in, 264–5
    utility of, 270–1
meats
    appropriate consumption of, 155–7
    cholesterol and, 270
    grass-fed, 250–1
    lunchmeats and, 234, 245
    processed, 152, 245, 269
    protein from, 146–8, 152–3
    section of grocery store, 244
    served as side dish, 156–7, 337
media
    eating habits and, 73
    influence on attitudes, 86–7
    perception of weight and, 52–3
Medical Myths, 42–7, 57–8, 149, 169, 195, 213, 406
meditation, 396–8
    practices, 399–402
menus, three-week, 368–70
milk
    children's consumption of, 170, 246, 307–8
    fat content of, 169, 233
    grass-fed cows and, 251
    healthy consumption of, 233–4, 247–8
    organic vs. regular, 247–8
mindfulness of breathing exercise, 400–1
mini-meditation, 399–400
moderation, 178–9
monounsaturated fats, 162–3, 319
motivation, for change in health habits, 20–4
muscle
    fat vs., 59–60
    protein and, 154–5
muscle-strengthening exercises, 376–7

National Association to Advance Fat Acceptance, 175
National Football League, exercise promotion by, 91
National Heart Lung and Blood Institute guidelines, 54–5
National Institute of Health, guidelines of, 55, 378
natural foods, organic foods vs., 249–50
natural remedies
    dangerous, 205–6
    realistic expectation for, 204–5
Nebuchadnezzar, 81
New American Plate, 108, 408
non-REM sleep, 112–13
nutrition
    carbohydrates and, 123–36, 138–40
    children's, 307–8, 312, 314
    entrenched habits and, 68–9, 164–5
    fast food and, 69, 73–4, 85, 258–9
    junk food and, 73–9

Index

moderation and, 178–9
nutritional content of food and, 73–9. See also food labels.
psychology of food and, 72–3
vitamins and supplements and, 195–6
nutrition labels. See food labels.
Nutritional Labeling and Education Act, 225
nuts
   healthy fats in, 285
   servings per week, 269

oatmeal, 282
Obama, Barack, 223
Obama, Michele, 89, 91
obesity
   "acceptance" of, 174–5
   Americans and, 88
   BMI and, 54–5
   childhood, 87–91
   diabetes and, 104
   excess glycogen storage and, 126–7
   family history of, 44–5
   high Glycemic Index foods and, 126
   measures of, 54–5
   overweight vs., 88
   real causes of, 60–2, 90
   risk of death from, 57–8
   social costs of, 92–3
   See also weight.
olive oil, 319
omega-3 fats
   fish sources of, 154, 163, 244, 267, 285
   grass-fed animals and, 251
   plant sources of, 163
omega-6 fats, sources of, 163

organic foods
   authenticity of, 250
   milk, 247–8
   natural foods vs., 249–50
   real value of, 248–9
overweight, obesity vs., 88. See also obesity.

pain, absence as health indicator, 42–4
pantry, home
   evaluating, 235–7
   foods to add to, 238–9
   food to eliminate from, 237
   restocking, 237–41
   shopping list for, 234
Paul of Tarsus, 11
peer pressure, health habits and, 177
Percent Daily Value, meaning of, 78–9
pesticides, in food, 247–50
physical education, 89
Pilates, 396
Pilates, Joseph, 396
Pinto, Rory, 398
PIYOLET, 396
polyunsaturated fats, 162–3
portion sizes,
   increasing, 407–8
   serving size and, 235, 254, 406–7
practicing what you preach, 13–14
prayers, mealtime, 410–11
pregnancy, gestational diabetes and, 103–4
preparation, for change, 22–3
prescription medications, lifestyle changes vs., 46–7
preservatives, in food, 247–8
processed meats, 152, 245, 269

protein
  appropriate consumption of, 151–3, 155–6
  amino acids and, 144–5, 147
  basic biology of, 144–5
  dairy as source of, 148
  deficiency of, 151
  dietary benefits of, 129
  fish as source of, 154
  glucose and, 130
  meat as source of, 146–8, 152–3
  muscle building and, 154–5
  overconsumption of, 149–50, 155
  shakes, 154–6
  sources of, 146–51, 151–2
  vegetable sources of, 149, 153
psyche, assessing, 21
push-up tests, 376

quinoa, 352–3

Recipe for Success Foundation, nutritional education and, 91
recipes
  breakfast, 280–290
    Buckwheat Blueberry Pancakes, 290
    Cherry Oatmeal, 282
    Crepe Ambrosia with Sauce Ala Orange, 283
    Granola, 288
    Power Bar, 287
    Sauce Ala Orange, 284
    Smoothie, 289
  brunch, 292–300
    Frittata, 299
    Mediterranean Latkes, 292
    One Pot Breakfast, 298
    Quesadilla Margherita, 297
    Roasted Garlic, 293
    Roasted Garlic Butter, 294
    Smoked Salmon Omelet, 295
    Tomato Relish, 296
    Turkey Pita with Tomato Relish, 296
  dinner, 332–41
    Almost Meatless Chili, 332
    Avocado Mousse, 338
    Blackened Catfish over Sautéed Spinach Topped with Mango Papaya Salsa, 336
    Chicken Ahuacatl, 338
    Ginger Tofu Fried Rice, 337
    Jasmine Jambalaya, 340
    Jerk Chicken, 335
    Johnny Cakes with Jerk Chicken, 334
    Leg of Lamb with Ratatouille, 333
    Mango Papaya Salsa, 336
    Pineapple Jicama Escabeche, 339
    Ratatouille, 333
    Salmon in Foil, 341
  grilled dishes, 360–3
    Beer Butt Chicken, 362
    Cajun Meatloaf Burger, 360
    Chimichurri Sauce, 363
    Grilled BBQ Veggies, 361
    Grilled Flank Steak, 363

Index

lunch, 306–15, 318–22, 324–30
  Bean Burrito, 321
  Black Eyed Pea Salad, 322
  Box Lunch Bagel, 314
  Bow Tie Pasta, 322
  Chilled Asparagus Soup, 322
  Couscous and Fruit Salad, 318
  Deconstructed Hard Boiled Egg Salad, 328
  Not Your Mama's BLT, 310
  Not Your Mama's BLT #4, 311
  Peanut Butter Tea Sandwiches, 306
  Pork of Shrimp Stir-Fry, 330
  Roasted Chicken Chopped Salad, 320
  Roasted Chicken Salad, 313
  Roasted Chicken Salad on a Bun, 313
  Roasted Garlic Vinaigrette, 320
  Roasted Sweet Potato Soup, 327
  Smoked Salmon Pizza, 319
  Somebody's Shrimp Boil, 325
  Texas Caviar, 322
  Tomato Soup Lite, 315
  Traditional Cocktail Sauce, 325
  Trail Mix Cracker, 307
  Turkey Sloppy Joe, 329
  snacks, 346–8
  Whole-Wheat Bagel Surprise, 348
salad dressings
  Honey-Citrus Mustard Dressing, 356
  Poppy Seed Vinaigrette, 356
  Sweet Onion Vinaigrette, 354
salads, 313, 318, 320, 322, 328, 350–6
  Black Eyed Pea Salad, 322
  Couscous and Fruit Salad, 318
  Deconstructed Hard Boiled Egg Salad, 328
  Organic Quinoa Salad, 352
  Panzanella Salad, 354
  Quinoa, 353
  Roasted Chicken Chopped Salad, 320
  Roasted Chicken Salad, 313
  Southwestern Cobb Salad, 355
  Spinach Salad, 350
  Waldorf with a Twist, 351
  key code to, 273
  meaning of terms in, 273
red meat
  appropriate consumption of, 155–7
  health risks of, 155
refined grains, 135–9
REM sleep, 112–13
respiratory disease, smoking and, 109

responsibility, personal, 47–8
restaurants
    doggy bags and, 259–60
    fast food, 258–9
    healthy eating at, 252–6
    upscale, 259
reverse osmosis water purification systems, 214–5
rice cookers, 340
Roth, MeMe, 91

Safe Drinking Water Act, 212
salad dressings
    recipes for, 320, 354–4
    unhealthy, 234–5
salads
    recipes for, 318, 320, 322, 328, 350–6
    restaurant, 256–8
salt. See sodium.
saturated fats
    chemistry of, 168
    daily value of, 228, 269–70
    foods high in, 169
    limiting intake of, 169
saving money, healthy eating and, 260, 264–5
school lunches, healthy, 302–3, 306–7
seeds, servings per week, 269
self-assessment, health, 12–13, 17–20, 23–4, 40–2, 62–4
self-centeredness, health and, 91–3
self-esteem
    developing healthy, 9–12
    overweight children and, 87
serving sizes
    food labels and, 229–30, 407
    portion control and, 235, 254, 406–7

shame, overcoming sense of, 10
shopping lists, grocery, 234, 242
simple carbohydrates, chemistry of, 124–5
sleep, getting adequate, 111–17
smoking
    cancer and, 105
    economic costs of, 92
    heart disease and, 100
    need to quit, 402
    not even in moderation, 178–9
    respiratory disease and, 109
sodium
    daily value of, 79, 267
    substitutes for, 298
solid calories, 191
soluble fibers, 128
spirituality, perspective on health of, 79–82
Standing Meditation, 401–2
starch, 126
Stevia, 365
Stokes, Sarah, 387
strokes
    basics of, 95–9
    diet and, 139
    symptoms of, 99
sugar
    beverages and, 268
    substitutes for, 365
    white, 365
    See also fructose and glucose.
supplements
    amino acids, 155
    appropriate uses of, 195, 197–8, 206–7
    dangerous, 205–6
    faddishness and, 194–5, 196–8

Index

protein, 154–5
realistic expectations for, 204–5
well-balanced diet vs., 195–6
See also vitamins.
Surles, Robert (Chef Bobo), 15–16, 73, 246–7, 409

Tabatsky, David, 310–11
table push-ups, 389
table squats, 391
tap water
bottled water vs., 212
pollutants in, 210–12
teenagers, health and, 93–5
television, perception of weight and, 52–3
Texas Commission on Environmental Quality tests, 211
thinness, health and 45–6
Thompson, William, 276
To Do List, 25–6, 418
tofu, protein from, 149
trans fats
development of, 165–6
health risks of, 166–7
margarine and, 246
prevalence of, 167–8
Trump, Donald, 27
Tupper, Earl, 343
Twinkies, nutritional content of, 75
type 1 diabetes, 102–3
type 2 diabetes, 88, 103, 139

Ungerleider, Lillian, 343–4
unsaturated fats
chemistry of, 162–3
health benefits of, 163
U.S. Department of Agriculture, 25, 184–5

U.S. Department of Health and Human Services, Dietary Guidelines for Americans, 139

vegan diets, 149, 153, 195, 329
vegetable chips, 326
vegetables
cancer prevention and, 107–8
including in children's diets, 299, 306–7
protein from, 149, 153
source of carbohydrates, 133–4
shopping for, 243
source of fiber, 127
vegetarian diets, 149, 153, 176–7, 195
vitamins
appropriate uses of, 195, 197–8, 206–7
faddishness and, 194–8
food sources of, 199–203
functions of, 199–203
realistic expectations for, 204–5
recommended daily allowances of, 199–203
well-balance diet vs., 195–6

water
adequate intake of, 210, 217
bottled, 212–14
filtered, 214–5
need for, 216–7
tap, 210–12
weight
appearance vs. healthy, 45–6
American obsession with, 52–3
ideal, 53–6

433

indicator of health, 54
muscle vs. fat and, 59–60
wrong focus on, 59–60
real causes of gaining, 60–1, 90
See also obesity.
weight lifting, 380
weight loss, science behind, 132–3, 189
white bread
breaking habit of, 244
nutritional value of, 136–9
White House Task Force on Childhood Obesity, 89

whole grains
breads, 134–5, 244
nutritional value of, 128, 133–6
servings per day, 267
Whopper, nutritional content of, 74
Wonder Bread, 136–9

Xylitol, 365

yoga, 394–5

About the Authors

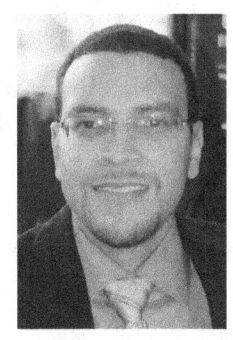

Randall Wright, MD is first and foremost a family man, committed to his wife and two children and the larger community that revolves around his church, neighborhood, and hospital clinic. Dr. Wright received a Bachelor of Science degree in Physics from Xavier University of Louisiana, a Bachelor of Electrical Engineering from Georgia Institute of Technology, and a medical doctorate degree from Emory University School of Medicine. He completed his internship at Louisiana State University and a residency at Baylor College of Medicine, with a fellowship in their Department of Neurology. Dr. Wright currently serves as the Medical Director of two centers in Houston, Texas: the Conroe Regional Neurovascular Stroke Center and the Stroke Care Unit at Health South Rehabilitation Hospital in the Woodlands. He also serves as the Director of Medical Subspecialties and Staff Neurologist at the Sadler Clinic.

Dr. Wright has won the Hospital Corporation of America (HCA) Frist Humanitarian Award for 2011 at Conroe Hospital for volunteer efforts in his community in regard to spreading the life saving message of healthy lifestyle change and for bringing state-of-the-art stroke care to a community hospital. Dr. Wright has established himself on the national stage through his continued work with the American Heart Association, first being named to Texas State Advocacy Committee in 2006, followed by his representing Texas at the national kick off of the Power to End Stroke Campaign. Dr. Wright was named an AHA Legacy Award winner in 2008. Through the AHA, he partnered with Gospel recording artist Kirk Franklin in 2009 to present the message of heart health to the city of Houston. He appeared on *Great Day Houston* and spoke about the signs and symptoms of stroke. That same year, the AHA recognized Dr. Wright as an outstanding member of the South Central Affiliate. In April 2010, Dr. Wright was once again featured on *Great Day Houston* to continue spreading the message of stroke prevention.

More recently, in 2011, he was asked to serve as Chairman of the Stroke Committee for the American Heart Association's Southwestern affiliate. In this role, Dr. Wright leads the fight against stroke across six states by setting AHA priorities for stroke care for hospitals, stroke legislation, and developing protocols for the stroke chain of survival in those states.

In Houston, Dr. Wright currently serves as Chairman of the Montgomery County American Heart Association, volunteers for the Speakers Bureau of the Houston Chapter of the Alzheimer's Association, and was a participant in the Leadership Houston Program.

Dr. Wright plays golf, enjoys jogging with his children, is an aspiring cook, and says, "I live my life according to Philippians 4:13."

About the Authors

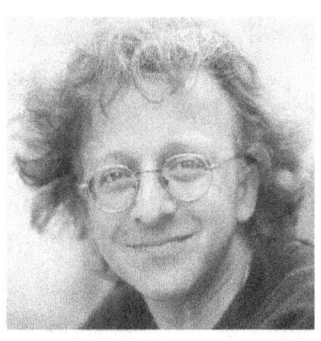

David Tabatsky is a writer, editor, teacher, director, and performing artist.

He received his Bachelor of Arts in Communications and a Masters in Theatre Education, both from Adelphi University in Garden City, New York.

David is the coauthor and editor of *The Cancer Book: 101 Stories of Courage, Support and Love*, from the Chicken Soup for the Soul series (2009). He is the coauthor, with Bruce Kluger, of *Dear President Obama: Letters of Hope from Children Across America* (2009). He has collaborated with Dr. Mark Banschick on *The Intelligent Divorce: Because Your Kids Come First* (Intelligent Book Press 2010 and 2011). David wrote *The Boy Behind the Door: How Salomon Kool Escaped the Nazis* (KTAV 2009). He was the Consulting Editor for Marlo Thomas and her *New York Times* bestseller *The Right Words at the Right Time, Volume 2: Your Turn* (2006). He has published two editions of *What's Cool Berlin*, a comic travel guide to Germany's capital, and has written for *The Forward, Parenting,* and *Sesame Street Parent,* among others. David currently works with Genentech USA, Inc., facilitating writing workshops *(Write To Fight Cancer)* at hospitals around the country.

David has worked professionally in theatre and circus as an actor, clown, and juggler, appearing in New York at Lincoln Center, Radio City Music Hall, the Beacon Theatre, and throughout the United States, Europe, Russia and Japan, including his critically acclaimed solo performance at the

Edinburgh Fringe Festival. He played a significant role in the resurgence of the *Variete* movement in Germany, with original shows at the *Chamaleon* in Berlin and the *Schmidt* in Hamburg, among others. He directed *Kinderzirkus Taborka* at the renowned Tempodrom in Berlin.

He has taught for the American School of London, die Etage in Berlin, the Big Apple Circus School, the United Nations International School, and the Cathedral of St. John the Divine. He serves on the theatre faculty at Adelphi University and is a teaching artist for the Henry Street Settlement with a focus on special education.

David lives in New York City with his children, Max and Stella.

Please visit www.tabatsky.com.

Order Form

The WRIGHT CHOICE

Your Family's Prescription For
HEALTHY EATING, MODERN
FITNESS, & SAVING MONEY

RANDY WRIGHT, MD
DAVID TABATSKY

By mail: InTouch Media Health Network USA,
P.O. Box 25410, Houston Texas 77265
By internet: www.drwrightrx.com

Quantity Book _____

SUBTOTAL _____

Shipping and Handling
USA: Shipping 5.95 + 1.00 Each Additional Book Free Shipping over 5 books
Canada: Shipping 9.95 + 2.00 Each Additional Book Free Shipping over 5 books
Europe: Shipping 14.95 + 4.00 Each Additional Book Free Shipping over 10 books

TOTAL _____

Payment method:
☐ Check/Money Order (payable to "InTouch Media Health Network USA" in US$ and drawn on a US Bank)
☐ Visa   ☐ Mastercard
☐ AMEX (Statement will reflect a charge to "InTouch Media Health Network")

Card No: _____

Exp. date: _____ Card Security Code _____ (Required)

Cardholder name (Print): _____

Card Signature: _____

Ship to: (Please use credit card statement address)

Name: _____

Address: _____

City, State, Zip: _____

Phone: _____ Email (optional): _____

Please visit

www.TheWrightChoiceRx.com

www.ingramcontent.com/pod-product-compliance
Lightning Source LLC
Chambersburg PA
CBHW071056230426
43666CB00009B/1729